A Woman's Concise Guide to Common Medical Tests

D0557689

20.2

A Woman's Concise Guide to Common Medical Tests

Michele C. Moore, M.D.
Caroline M. de Costa, M.D.

Rutgers University Press
New Brunswick, New Jersey, and London

Library of Congress Cataloging-in-Publication Data

Moore, Michele.
A woman's concise guide to common medical tests / Michele C. Moore,
Caroline M. De Costa.
       p. cm.
   Includes bibliographical references and index.
   ISBN 0–8135–3579–4 (hardcover : alk. paper) — ISBN
0–8135–3580–8 (pbk. : alk. paper)
      1. Diagnosis—Popular works.   2. Medical screening—Popular works.
3. Periodic health examinations—Popular works.   4. Women—Health
and hygiene—Popular works.   I. De Costa, Caroline, 1947–   II. Title.
   RC71.3.M665 2005
   618.1′075—dc22

                                                            2004016426

A British Cataloging-in-Publication record for this book is available from
the British Library.

Manufactured in the United States of America

Contents

Acknowledgments

We wish to thank Audra Wolfe, Adi Hovav, and Marilyn Campbell at Rutgers University Press for their ongoing support during the production of this book. Also our agent Sally Brady for her guidance, Dr. Tim Elston for his input into the chapter on breast screening, and Javed de Costa and Josie Valese for advice on the finer points of word processing. The staff of Cairns Base Hospital library continued to produce every article requested with their usual alacrity and patience. And our families were as helpful as ever—we thank them all.

Disclaimer

We also thank the women whose stories we've borrowed. Their names and circumstances have been changed and sometimes blended to preserve their privacy.

A Woman's Concise Guide to Common Medical Tests

Introduction

Frannie Morris, a good-looking woman of about thirty-five, walked into our consulting office one day and announced that she wanted to know why she came in every year for a physical exam and certain tests. She knew she was supposed to come, but no one had ever explained the why and wherefore. She knew the information was probably somewhere on the Internet, but she didn't know exactly what she was looking for or how to interpret what she read. It was frustrating; no doctor had ever taken time to explain it to her fully, nor had the women's magazines addressed the question in a comprehensive manner.

Why do we doctors suggest physical checkups and certain tests? Is it to pay our office overhead costs and provide a reliable source of well patients? Is it habit, ingrained by custom? Or is there a rationale for all this?

The exams and tests are screening procedures that allow us to identify disease or potential problems at an early and more treatable or preventable stage. Yes, it is nice to see well people in our offices, but this is not the driving force behind our recommendations. Nor is it financial . . . in fact, treating illness is usually more financially productive than preventive care.

Who are we? We are two women physicians (we have the same "equipment" as you do) who met at medical school in Dublin, Ireland, and then went our separate ways for many years. Caroline returned to Australia to specialize in obstetrics and gynecology and, in the process, to birth and raise seven children. Michele returned to the United States to become a family practitioner specializing in women's health (that same equipment again) and to raise two children. Of course, husbands were also involved and supportive. We have a combined experience of almost sixty years of caring for women.

In our work with women, we have addressed questions like those of Frannie many times, and from this has evolved our journey as authors. Almost all of our writing has been in response to patients' questions alerting us to women's needs for in-depth answers to their questions. While the stories included in this book, and even the names of Frannie, her family, and friends are entirely fictitious, the concerns and questions raised are very real. Any resemblance to actual persons is coincidental.

So, to answer Frannie's original question, the physical exam that we do—including the history we take and the tests that accompany the exam—is a form of screening for illness or potential problems. These tests are for illnesses or conditions that exist in the present, but are currently causing no symptoms, and these are the tests we describe more fully for you in this book. We also talk about screening tests for conditions or problems that may occur in the future, tests that are possible because of advances in genetics technology.

The history that you give your doctor about events, medical and otherwise, that may have occurred in the intervening time between preventive care visits also gives clues to things that may endanger your health. The same is true of the physical exam. One easy example is that your doctor may notice a spot on your skin that could turn into skin cancer if not caught in time or even a full-blown skin cancer that you hadn't noticed.

We talk about all these different tests and procedures, and we explain why we recommend doing them, what they are intended to achieve, as well as their limitations. In addition, we give you details of some of the more common tests performed in conjunction with a routine office visit—these are diagnostic tests, concerned with the diagnosis of a particular symptom or complaint, rather than screening tests; but because they are common, we feel they have a place in this book.

In the last chapter, we visit the more positive side of preventive care: not looking for early signs of disease, but describing the things that you can do to optimize your health. Indeed, whole books are available on this topic, making it possible for you to spend all your time implementing the suggestions. But we think you are probably too busy for that and have boiled it down to a practical, health-promoting regimen. We also keep the book reasonably brief for the same reasons. At the end of each chapter, and at the end of the book, we have listed other sources of information—both written and on the Internet—to help you do further research, if desired. And in our final chapter, we give you some clues about how to use and interpret health information, especially that available on the Internet. We hope you find this book is a resource that you can consult frequently to supplement and explain other information you may have found or been given by your health care providers.

Every woman, including doctors, is a daughter; and as our mothers age, they need our assistance more and more in understanding medical care that is growing increasingly complex. As everyone ages, trusted physicians also retire and people are forced to make new connections with new providers. Trusting strangers can be difficult and young and old alike often need help traversing this minefield of new medical relationships and procedures. Remember that your mother has never been this age before, either. Our aim is to help you keep yourself and your loved ones as healthy as possible!

1 *What Is a Screening Test?*

Before talking about individual tests, it is important for us to explain just what we mean by *screening* and the difference between *screening* tests and *diagnostic* tests in health care.

A screening test is applied to a large group of people who appear to be well in order to detect problems before the person is aware of any symptoms and thereby to treat or head off these problems before they become serious. One of the best and most successful examples of a screening test is the Pap smear, which is designed to pick up early changes in cells scraped from the skin of the cervix, changes that if left alone might develop into cervical cancer.

A screening test or procedure is not intended to give each individual woman a diagnosis that is 100 percent accurate every time. Developed in the 1950s, the Pap smear is one of the most successful screening tools ever invented, and it continues to sharply reduce cervical cancer deaths in the United States and elsewhere. Yet it is not 100 percent accurate. Results with margins of 5 percent, false positive or false negative, are considered acceptable in all Pap screening programs. (We explain these terms, false positives and false negatives, in just a moment.) The intent of a screening test is simply *to give a fairly high probability that the disease or condition being screened for is or is not there.* If a screening test is positive, and it seems that the condition *may* be present, further tests are done to reach a definite diagnosis. If the screening test is negative, no further action will be taken immediately, but a further screening test will be done at some recommended time interval—for example, in the United States, Paps are recommended about every three years, after an initial series of three consecutive normal smears have been done at yearly intervals. Having the test done regularly increases the chances of picking up changes early; even if a positive result is missed once it is likely to be found the next time. We explain this as we go along.

Let's be clear, too, that a screening test is not a *treatment* for a disease or condition. Having a Pap smear does not by itself reduce your chances of having cervical cancer, the test simply finds it early so it can be treated; likewise having a mammogram does not reduce your chances of having breast cancer, it simply picks up abnormalities earlier. Understanding the differences between screening tests and treatment is important: mistaken expectations have led to unnecessary disillusionment with some screening tests.

A diagnostic test is one that tells us whether or not the suspected disease is definitely present. This type of test is done to find the cause of a particular symptom or to follow up on a positive screening test. An good example is a *colposcopy* (examination of the cervix with a telescope) and biopsy of the cervix done for a woman with a positive Pap smear, or a breast biopsy done after a mammogram (screening test) indicating the suspicion of breast cancer. A diagnostic test, or series of such tests, is also done if you go to the doctor complaining of specific symptoms. An example is the urine test that is done if you complain of pain when you urinate.

A screening test needs to be both highly *sensitive* and highly *specific*. What do we mean by these terms? Being specific means that people identified by the test as being free of the disease or condition actually are free of that disease or condition. Being sensitive means it is highly probable that people who have the disease or condition will be identified by the test. However, as we've already mentioned, most screening tests are not 100 percent sensitive or specific, and so some false positive and false negative results will always occur with any screening test.

A *false positive* means that the test is positive in a person subsequently found not to have the disease in question. This is troublesome because it causes unfounded fear and anxiety, as well as the trauma and cost of further testing. In small percentages this is generally considered an acceptable risk. We'll be discussing false positives for most of the screening tests we describe. The implications vary in different conditions. For example, a false positive Pap smear may lead to a colposcopy and a biopsy (a small sample of tissue) being removed from the cervix. This is an uncomfortable procedure and can be distressing, but has no worrying long-term consequences. A suspicious shadow on a mammogram, however, may lead to a breast biopsy or even to more major surgery (see chapter 5 on breast screening). Clearly the implications here are much greater for a woman eventually found not to have a cancer. We believe you have a right to know about the false positive aspects of any screening test, so that you can make an informed decision before you agree to have one. At the same time, do be aware that the vast majority of screening tests have been clearly shown to reduce the incidence (in the population as a whole) of the conditions they are designed to detect.

A *false negative* occurs when the screening test does not pick up disease that is present. An example of this is a fecal occult blood test for colon cancer that is found to be negative for the presence of blood, even though the person is found to have colon cancer on other testing such as a colonoscopy. In this case, the test may have been done at a time when the cancer wasn't bleeding or it may have been a nonbleeding cancer. We don't expect screening tests to be 100 percent perfect, but we do expect them to give us a bit more of an advantage over disease than we would have without them. The implications of false negatives, of missing a serious condition, are believed to be reduced by testing regularly; for example, in the case of colon cancer screening, testing for people at risk is recommended yearly.

There are a few other requirements for a good screening test. It should be safe and minimally invasive. It makes no sense to screen whole segments of the population with tests that are apt to cause a whole bagful of problems in some, if not many, individuals. Tests should not present major risks to those being screened. If there are risks, they should be clearly explained beforehand so that you can decide for yourself whether or not you want to take the test. For instance, a small percentage of people who have a colonoscopy to check for early signs of colon cancer may encounter perforation of the bowel, a complication requiring major surgery to correct. Most people, informed of this risk in advance, consider it a small price to pay for the security of knowing they don't have colon cancer—but you do need to know, and have time to think about, the implications for yourself should this uncommon complication happen to you.

A screening test should also be relatively inexpensive. Again, the medical community can't justify a very expensive test to screen large populations when the expected outcome is to pick up only a few people who may be positive and then subject them to further diagnostic tests. In the real world, screening must be cost effective. "Cost" includes not only the monetary cost of running the test itself, but also the cost of investigating everyone with abnormal results. If there are an unduly high number of falsely positive or negative tests, the cost will be unjustifiably high.

Many national organizations and institutions are concerned with assessing all types of screening tests and making recommendations about their use and availability—more about this later in this chapter. The National Taskforce on Preventive Care (a group of experts convened by the U.S. Public Health Services) is one such body that assesses and makes recommendations for and against a wide range of screening tests. One of the factors that obviously must be considered in making their recommendations is cost.

It also doesn't make much sense to screen for illnesses if there is no treatment or prevention to offer once the illness is detected. Here again, the Pap smear is a good example of an effective screening test because through Pap screening, most cervical problems are treated before they ever have a chance to progress to a full-blown cancer. On the other hand, we don't currently screen people for lung cancer—even heavy smokers—with routine chest X-rays: it has been shown to make no difference to the course of the illness.

A screening test also relies on the disease in question developing slowly enough so that the problem can be detected with screening and then treated effectively. Again, cervical cancer provides an ideal disease model to illustrate the value of screening tests: it takes some years to develop from the early changes, which can be found on Pap smears.

In this book we deal extensively with screening for cancers of the cervix, breast, and colon, as well as for heart disease and diabetes—all of which are major health concerns for women. We then go on to cover other forms of screening and some diagnostic tests. Although we don't aim to give comprehensive information about the diseases, we do direct you to reliable sources where such information can be found.

Recommendations for screening may differ from one country to another; even within countries, recommendations may even differ between states or provinces. When we talk about Pap screening, for example, you'll see that the recommended time between tests varies among the United States, the United Kingdom, and Australia. Where there are several national bodies concerned with a particular disease or condition there may also be differences of opinion about what tests should be offered and how often. Both the American Cancer Society and the American College of Obstetricians and Gynecologists have a strong interest in preventing cervical cancer, but the wording of their recommendations for Pap smears differs slightly. Overall, however, a general consensus has emerged as to the value and importance of screening. Regional differences in opinion, within countries as well as between them, may reflect differences in the incidence rates for various diseases and conditions in various places, or perhaps the ability of the country's health service to pay for tests, but they do not usually imply big differences in standards of health care.

In different countries, and also at different times of a woman's life, there may be different methods of paying for screening tests. In the United Kingdom and Australia, for example, there are free national Pap smear and mammogram screening tests at intervals approved by government health departments. In the United States there is tremendous variance in health insurance programs. Many screening tests are covered by health insurance programs at no additional charge, although some tests are provided free of charge, or free at specific times, such as mammograms in Breast Cancer Awareness Month. Since insurance coverage programs vary dramatically in the United States, American women should be sure to check their program allowances. You may need a referral from your doctor before scheduling appointments or appearing for tests. Be sure to call your insurance company if you have questions. We'll deal with these matters more specifically in individual chapters.

In real life, many women start having routine screenings through the encouragement of family and friends. To make this book more interesting for you and to give examples you can more easily relate to, we have followed the family and friends of Frannie Morris as they encounter the need to take a variety of screening tests. Although drawn from the histories of the many women we have cared for as patients, the Morrises and their friends are fictional characters. Frannie's is a typical American extended family with a melding of many genetic pools and traditions and their friends also have a wide range of backgrounds. We feel that their experiences of health and health care systems, as we describe them for you, are typical of many Americans'.

Every year, the Morris family and its extended alliances meet at the home of Royal and Jean Morris for Thanksgiving dinner. Royal's sister Rachel and her family and Jean's sister Beverly and her family are always included. This has been a twenty-five-year tradition. Last year, the women started talking about health care while in the kitchen heating all their favorite foods and filling platters to take to the table. Lots more talking and joking than work was going on—all part of the fun of the annual event. Jean and Beverly were reminiscing about Gran, their mother, as they decorated the potato salad made from her recipe. Gran's potato salad graced every family dinner party, even with turkey and all the trimmings.

Rachel always brought her acclaimed pies to family events, but she was recently diagnosed with diabetes and her statement, "Well, girls, next year somebody else will have to take over the pies," led the talk from food to health matters. She said that her diagnosis made her more aware that all of us should be checked for various health problems so that we can take care of them early.

"Yeah, Rachel, I guess that means Jean and I should be lining up for that colon test you hear about. After all, Gran did die of colon cancer." This comment came from Beverly, the family pragmatist.

"Yes, and we should do the usual stuff—Pap smears and all."

By the end of the evening, the women had made an informal pact with one another to begin doing all the preventive care available to them, starting with the New Year, and agreed that they would give each other any and all support needed.

Who are the Morris women?

Frannie Morris was our first contact with the family. Frannie is a young (mid thirties) divorced mother of two. She has all the stresses of a working mother added to single parenthood. Sometimes, she feels that she has no time or energy to take care of herself after dealing with all the other demands on her time.

Jean Morris is Frannie's mother. She is postmenopausal and is dealing with issues connected with aging and seeing friends stricken by illness. She and Beverly Acton are sisters, and they share a family risk of both colon cancer and heart disease. Gran, their mother, died of colon cancer at age sixty-seven, which seems quite young to them now. Pop, their father, died from a heart attack at the age of sixty, having suffered from hypertension (high blood pressure) for many years.

Rachel Morris Rice is Frannie's aunt, sister to Frannie's dad, Royal. Rachel has always been pleasingly plump. She and Royal are Native American, members of the Mohawk tribe of northern New York State. Rachel, Jean, and Beverly are contemporaries and have been close friends since college.

Janine is Rachel Morris's daughter and is about to go off to college. She is an attractive and bright teenager, but has not been very physically active in the past few years.

Hannah Harris Acton is married to Beverly Acton's son Jeff, Frannie's cousin. Hannah wants to have a baby for Jeff, even though she will be an older mother. She has two children by a previous marriage and Jeff is wonderful with them.

You will also meet a few of the friends with whom these women share their particular problems. We hope that discussing medical tests from the points of view of these typical women will help to make the situations and the need for screening real to you.

Resources

Throughout this book we give you details of websites and other books you can access for more information. The appendix includes a table of basic screening tests recommended at different ages. In chapter 17, we also give some advice on how to assess what you read on the Internet. Because information can be posted there without undergoing the same kind of scrutiny that book publishers require, it may be biased or just plain wrong. We tell you how to separate the reliable from the not so reliable, and how to apply the information you read to your own situation.

WEBSITES WITH GENERAL INFORMATION ABOUT SCREENING TESTS

The U.S. Preventive Services Task Force is a panel of experts that evaluates the latest scientific evidence on preventive measures in health care. Their website is at *www.ahcpr.gov* and has a comprehensive alphabetical list of test recommendations for a wide range of conditions. The Task Force panel applies very strict criteria when considering scientific evidence; and in some cases you may find that they do not accept certain screening or other tests that other national bodies have endorsed. This is part of the nature of medical and health care practice. If you are concerned about that fact that slightly different views are being expressed about a condition you or a loved one faces, we suggest you discuss your individual situation with your doctor.

Four organizations have excellent websites that dealing with the entire range of cancers. Information found on them includes not only screening tests, but also early detection, diagnosis, statistics, and treatment, as well as where to find help in your area. All four sites are highly recommended sources of up-to-date, accurate, and useful information.

- www.cancer.org is the website of the American Cancer Society.
- *www.cancernet.nci.nih.gov* is the information site of the National Cancer Institute.
- *www.cancer.gov/publications* gives information about specific cancers and how to find help in your local area. You can telephone the U.S. Cancer Information Service at 1–800–4–CANCER.
- *www.obgyn.net* is one of the websites of MedSpecialties.com and is designed to provide information to the public. It also

lists all certified specialist obstetricians/gynecologists in the United States.

BOOKS

The books listed here cover a broad range of screening and other medical tests. Books dealing with specific topics are listed at the ends of the appropriate chapters.

Buckman, Robert and others. *What You Really Need to Know about Cancer.* Baltimore: Johns Hopkins University Press, 1997.

Moore, Michele C., and Caroline M. de Costa. *Do You Really Need Surgery? A Sensible Guide to Hysterectomy and Other Procedures for Women.* New Brunswick, NJ: Rutgers University Press, 2004.

Segen, Joseph, and Joseph Stauffer. *The Patient's Guide to Medical Tests: Everything You Need to Know about the Tests Your Doctor Prescribes.* New York: Facts on File, Inc., 1998.

Zaret, Barry, ed. *The Yale University School of Medicine Patient's Guide to Medical Tests.* Boston: Houghton Mifflin, 1997.

While increasing your knowledge about health care options is highly desirable and something we strongly encourage, it is best to discuss the information you find with your own doctor, particularly before taking any action, such as making a decision for or against surgery. What you find on the Internet or by reading a book (even our books!) may not apply to your own situation. You are an individual and deserve the personal care only your doctor can provide, in conjunction with the best treatment medical science can offer.

2 The Annual Physical Exam

Before Frannie Morris came to the office for her scheduled physical exam—or checkup—she received a patient questionnaire to fill out. This questionnaire asked about many potential areas of risk, as well as her personal and family health history. A copy of a sample questionnaire is in the appendix.

A patient questionnaire, or, when we all had more time, the face-to-face interview, does much to identify possible areas of susceptibility to illness. The seemingly meaningless chat with the doctor prior to your exam gives a lot of information about things that have happened since your last visit that may have added a new dimension to your risk profile. Frannie, for instance, a divorced mother of two young children, is dating again. This is not just a piece of social news—there are possible health ramifications. But more about that later.

When you are first ushered from the waiting room to the exam room, a series of small events takes place: the nurse takes your weight, height, blood pressure, pulse, temperature, and respiratory rate. Many people view these as unnecessary small annoyances, but they are actually low-tech, cost-effective screening tests.

An unexplained change in weight of ten pounds or more can be a signal to look for diseases like cancer or hormone disturbances.

A loss of height is often the first clue to bone disease, especially osteoporosis. This is responsible for much personal suffering, as well as an increasing financial burden on the health care system.

Blood pressure checks are responsible for the detection of one of the most common and quiet illnesses: hypertension. There is no better screening tool than the simple blood pressure cuff (sphygmomanometer) in the hands of a trained health care professional. High blood pressure is a contributor to heart attack, stroke, and probably dementia. It is usually silent, that is, without symptoms, and can be detected by this simple two-minute test.

Frannie asked and was told that her blood pressure was 120/80 — nice and normal — which was welcome news because high blood pressure runs in Frannie's family. And what is normal? It is generally accepted that any blood pressure under 140/90 is normal, although in a young person, this blood pressure reading may be qualified as borderline. Recently, readings above 130/80, but below 140/90, have been classified as pre-hypertensive. Low blood pressure is rarely a cause for concern in healthy people; many young women consistently have low blood pressure readings.

Your pulse can give us a clue to heart problems: if your pulse is too high (over 100 beats per minute), too low (under 60 beats per minute in a non-athletic person), or if the beat is irregular in any way, we follow up with an EKG. Frannie's pulse was in the 90s because she always feels nervous when she visits a doctor!

For screening purposes, respiratory rate (number of breaths per minute) and temperature aren't as useful as screens in healthy people because abnormalities are usually temporary and accompanied by symptoms of overt illness, such as a flu, another infectious disease, or a lung condition, such as asthma. In other words, you know you are ill and are not being screened for unknown disease.

After the nurse took Frannie's vital signs, Dr. Hatch entered the exam room and sat on the little stool across from Frannie.

Since Dr. Hatch is new to the practice, she carefully reviewed Frannie's patient questionnaire and asked Frannie to tell her more about the family history of heart disease and colon cancer. She also asked many questions about Frannie's social circumstances: Was she currently sexually active and, if so, was she using condoms? How was she managing the demands of work and single parenting? Did she have adequate support systems? Frannie hadn't thought of these things as impacting her health, but of course, they do. Frannie told the doctor about her close-knit and very supportive family.

After Dr. Hatch was satisfied that she had covered all the possible trouble areas ascertainable by history, she instructed Frannie to change into a gown and left the room to give Frannie privacy.

A few minutes later, Dr. Hatch returned and began the physical exam. She had already looked at Frannie in a general way and had noted that Frannie was a well-nourished and well-developed woman who looked neither older nor younger than her stated age of thirty-five. She ran her fingers through Frannie's hair and over her scalp, feeling for the texture of the hair and for any skin lesions on the scalp. She probed down into the neck, feeling for lumps or bumps that shouldn't be there, and felt for the thyroid gland, which lies like a butterfly over the front of the throat and is not normally easily palpable. In this process, she was also forming an impression of the texture of Frannie's skin and looking at it for acne or other skin diseases. By the end of the exam, she had looked at Frannie's skin all over, searching for anything indicative of an early cancerous or precancerous lesion.

Next, Dr. Hatch looked in Frannie's ears, throat, and nose. These are part of a general physical exam, but they rarely yield any unsuspected problems since symptoms usually signal problems in these areas. She looked in Frannie's eyes with an ophthalmoscope, an instrument used in viewing the layers of the eye, including the optic nerve and blood vessels at the back.

All doctors are not equally skilled in this part of the exam, but in experienced hands, early changes due to high blood pressure, diabetes, or a host of other diseases can be recognized. If your doctor is not especially skilled in this exam, she will be more likely to refer you to an optometrist or ophthalmologist for eye exams. This is a good idea anyway if you are older than forty. Prior to the exam with the ophthalmoscope, Dr. Hatch shined a light in Frannie's eyes and watched to see if the pupils responded, if they responded symmetrically in both eyes, and if the eyes could move symmetrically through their range of movement. When she had looked in Frannie's throat, she had noted that the uvula (the little wormlike structure hanging down from the palate) moved symmetrically when Frannie said "Ah." Also, Frannie's tongue moved equally well to the left and right. Though these procedures may seem silly, they actually demonstrate that the cranial nerves (from the brain) responsible for these movements are intact. So, in fact, they are good basic screening for neurological illnesses.

Moving on down the torso, the next stop on the physical exam was the breast exam. First, Dr. Hatch looked at Frannie's breasts, checking to see whether they hung symmetrically and were free of any dimpled skin or obvious lumps. Then she gently felt each breast with the flat surface of her fingers, checking for any lumps or areas of abnormal thickening under her fingers. She also examined Frannie's armpits to be sure there were no lymph nodes or swollen glands. Contented with the normal findings, she murmured, "Good, good," after inspecting each breast.

Next, the stethoscope came out. Some old doctors' signs state "Two cents extra for the tubes," referring to the stethoscope, the high-tech medicine of its day! And in fact, despite advances in technology, the stethoscope is still an essential medical tool. Dr. Hatch listened carefully to Frannie's heart and lungs. Again, it's unusual to find anything wrong in the lungs of a healthy person with no complaints. Auscultation (the medical term for a listening) of the heart can sometimes reveal sounds in addition to the normal "lub-dup" that doctors listen for, sounds that may need follow-up tests. Frannie was reassured that her heart sounded normal.

Before hanging the stethoscope out of the way, Dr. Hatch listened to Frannie's abdomen, to hear the bowel sounds. The bowel makes a slight gurgling sound, like water going down a drain. Satisfied that Frannie's bowels sounded quite normal, Dr. Hatch gently touched all over her stomach, feeling for tenderness, involuntary tightening of the stomach wall muscles, and any abnormal masses or organs. Conditions such as an enlarged liver can be detected in this way. While she was in the area, Dr. Hatch felt Frannie's femoral pulses, which are in the groin, where the belly and thigh meet. She also felt the pulses in Frannie's legs to make sure that both sides were full and equal. She gently pinched Frannie's toes to observe how quickly the pink color returned, indicating the health of the peripheral (distant) circulation.

Next came the tap of a little red rubber hammer on Frannie's knees and ankles, in the crook of her elbows, and behind the point of her elbows; the resulting twitches were brisk and equal on both sides. This test was another part of the general screening of the nervous system.

So far, this exam was a bit more detailed than Frannie was accustomed to. However, Dr. Hatch believes that a woman's annual visit for her Pap smear and breast exam may be her only exposure to preventive health care and the examination should be as thorough as possible.

For the pelvic part of the exam, Dr. Hatch pulled out the stirrups on the exam table and had Frannie position her heels in the stirrups with her bottom scooted down to the end of the table. She placed a drape cloth, or modesty sheet, over Frannie's lap and had Frannie spread her legs apart. With the beam of a lamp directed at Frannie's crotch, Dr. Hatch looked carefully at the skin of Frannie's vulva, as she carefully parted the lips (labia). Then she took a speculum and gently slipped it into Frannie's vagina.

The speculum is an instrument specially designed to show the cervix, or neck, of the uterus (womb) that looks very much like a duck's bill with a handle. (If you are having your first Pap smear exam, you might like to ask your doctor or nurse to show you the instrument before it is used.) Dr. Hatch opened the blades (duck-bills) of the speculum so that she could see Frannie's cervix. As Frannie knew from previous experience, this was a bit uncomfortable, but not painful, and she could tell herself it would be over in a minute or two. In the center of the cervix, which feels like the end of your nose if you stick your finger far up into your vagina, is a small opening. It is through this opening that menstrual fluids pass and that sperm may enter the uterus and Fallopian tubes. To take Frannie's Pap smear, Dr. Hatch inserted a little brush that looked like a bottle brush into the cervix opening; she then made a half circle turn with the brush, after which she made a similar motion with a wooden or plastic spatula, ensuring that she obtained adequate cells for the Pap smear (more about this later). Because Frannie had just begun dating again and had had a few sexual experiences that may not have been "safe sex," Dr. Hatch also took a sample for chlamydia and gonorrhea testing.

Dr. Hatch removed the speculum from Frannie's vagina and inserted two lubricated, gloved fingers. She placed the other hand on Frannie's abdomen and between her two hands, Dr. Hatch felt for Frannie's uterus, tubes, and ovaries. She then inserted one finger into Frannie's anus and explained that she was feeling for the integrity of the wall between the vagina and the rectum, as well as checking for any problems around the anus itself.

After she finished the exam, Dr. Hatch excused herself for a few minutes, allowing Frannie time to dress. When the doctor returned, she told Frannie that the exam was normal, with no abnormal findings. A few simple screening blood tests were in order, not because of any suspicions aroused by the exam, but simply because of Frannie's age and family history. She ordered a complete blood count, commonly called a CBC, and a lipid profile to check on the blood fats. (See chapter 16 for details.) Since there was colon cancer in Frannie's family, Dr. Hatch suggested that Frannie do the fecal occult blood test, a test that is routinely done at a somewhat older age. She also explained that blood tests could be done to screen for syphilis and HIV, and were probably a good idea since Frannie had had a couple of episodes of unprotected sex. All of Frannie's tests were scheduled for the following week, so that Frannie could fast for the lipid test.

For women, the physical exam doesn't vary greatly with age—at least, past childhood—but the follow-up tests and procedures do vary according to age and the probability of various illnesses. You will see the correlation as we go through the various screens and compare them in the table of age-related screening tests in the appendix.

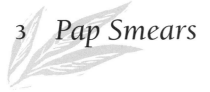

3 Pap Smears

We've freely referred to Pap smears, and, in a general way, they are common knowledge. Still, it's important to know a lot more about the Pap: its history, how it is taken, and how it helps you. The purpose of a Pap smear is to detect early abnormal changes in cells covering the cervix (the "neck" of the uterus or womb, found at the top of the vagina)—changes that, if left alone, might develop into cancer.

These changes are generally referred to as CIN, or cervical intra-epithelial neoplasia, a long term best summarized as "precancerous." CIN does not always progress to cancer, but because of the potential to do so, it is customary to assess and treat these precancerous changes. We know that Pap smear screening programs have greatly reduced the incidence of cervical cancer where they have been instituted. In the United States, most women who develop cervical cancer have either never had a Pap smear or have not had one for five years or more.

So what exactly is done when a Pap smear is taken? First of all, as Dr. Hatch did with Frannie, we need to visualize the cervix. This is why we use those funny-looking instruments (remember the bill of a duck?) to open your vagina so that we can see inside. If you have had the exam, we hope you found that it doesn't hurt, although we doubt that any woman thinks of it as fun. In certain situations, passing the instrument (the speculum) into the vagina may actually be painful. For example, breast-feeding women or postmenopausal women with low estrogen levels and thin vaginal skin may experience discomfort. Vaginal infection, such as candida (yeast), can also make the speculum insertion painful. Your doctor or nurse should be aware of these potential problems from your pre-exam conversation. If your physician forgets to ask about these issues, don't hesitate to mention any concerns you have well before "assuming the position." And if you have found the exam painful previously, speak up and tell your doctor or nurse this time. Nobody knowingly wants to hurt you; it may be that a smaller size or different type of speculum is more appropriate for you.

A Pap smear is the first thing we do when we examine your pelvis because we don't want anything, including our examining fingers, to disturb the cells of the cervix before we collect a good sample. The examiner should be well qualified and experienced in looking at the cervix because your cervix is as distinctive as your face. The examiner needs to recognize when to delay taking a smear. For example, if too much blood is still present from a recent period, or if obvious inflammatory changes should first be treated, the exam should be postponed. If that rare (thank goodness), obvious cauliflower-looking cervical cancer is on the cervix, the Pap may not be done at all.

When all systems are go, and your most intimate parts are adequately illuminated, the nurse or doctor will insert a tiny brush into the opening of your cervix. Alternatively, or in adjunct, she may use a small wooden or plastic scraper (spatula) to scrape cells from the cervix, especially from what is called the "squamocolumnar junction" which is where the inner and outer skin of the cervix meet (sort of like where the two textures of your inner and outer lips meet). It is important to obtain cells from this junction because it is the source of most cervical cancers. When the results of the Pap smear are reported, the lab routinely lets the doctor know whether or not cells from this junction are present by noting "endocervical cells present" or "absent." If cells are not present, the doctor will make a clinical judgment about repeating the test. In a pregnant woman, we usually use just the scraper, lest we inadvertently disturb the pregnancy.

While the cells on the brush or scraper are still moist, we immediately either spread them on a slide and spray them with a fixative to stop any changes from air exposure, or swish them off the brush or scraper into a liquid medium. If the latter process is used, the liquid is centrifuged (spun rapidly in a special machine) later, at the lab, and the cells are concentrated before being spread on a slide and dried. Many experts think this method gives a better sample, but it is slightly more expensive. Called ThinPrep, or liquid-based cytology, it is rapidly becoming the standard of care in private practice in the United States. Once the slides are prepared by either method, an expert cytotechnologist examines them under a microscope. "A what?" you say. A cytotechnologist is a laboratory technician who has been specially trained to look at the cells and identify any abnormalities. Many labs also utilize computer-assisted methods of scanning slides to reduce the inevitable percentage of human errors. Of course, improperly prepared slides also contribute to error, but many of these are recognized by the cytotechnologist. In a well-run lab, cytotechnologists have a set maximum number of slides that are to be read during a work shift, since fatigue is a large contributor to human error. In many areas, setting workload numbers like this is a condition for laboratory licensing.

After the cytotech reads your Pap smear, she reports the results in language that has been agreed upon by all labs to have a standard meaning. Because of this standardized nomenclature, Caroline can look at test results faxed to her in Australia from Michele in New Mexico and be able to interpret the results as well as she could if they had been done in the lab beside her consulting rooms.

The most common result is a straightforward normal or negative. In other words, the technician has viewed an adequate sample of cells and they are all normal in appearance.

What Is a Pap Smear?

- A Pap smear is a sample of cells taken from the surface of the cervix using a wooden or plastic spatula, some form of small brush, or both.
- The smear should contain cells from both the inside (endocervix) and the outside (ectocervix). This shows that the right part of the cervix has been sampled.
- The sample, containing cells mixed with mucus, is thinly smeared on a glass slide and is sprayed with a fixative to keep the cells intact.
- In the lab, a trained cytotechnologist (cyto = cell) examines the slide under a microscope, looking for cells that he or she knows from experience are abnormal.
- The cytologist decides whether the smear is satisfactory, i.e., enough cells can be easily seen, and if it is, then grades the smear.
- Automated devices are also used to check Pap smears; many labs now do a double check.
- The purpose of Pap smears is to pick up changes early, to treat them so they do not progress to cancer.

A report stating that the cells are negative for malignancy, but have benign reactive or inflammatory changes, is slightly less than normal. This is basically a normal Pap smear—the operative words are "negative for malignancy"—but with possible infection or hormonal changes affecting the cells. Your doctor may tell you not to worry or may treat whatever is causing the inflammation.

Definite abnormalities may be reported as showing or suggesting CIN—which is shorthand for saying cervical intra-epithelial neoplasia. This literally means changes or "new growth" within the cells. As these changes progress and become more extreme, the cells more clearly resemble cancer cells.

CIN 1 can be regarded as a mild change. CIN 2 is moderate, and CIN 3 indicates severe changes. These alterations are still within the cell itself and are not cancer as such. They are, however, changes that are likely to progress to cancer if they are not treated.

Different Terms Used to Describe Your Pap Smear

Pap smears report changes in cells that may progress into cancer. Only very rarely does an abnormal Pap mean that cancer has actually developed.

Normal or negative. Most Pap reports have this result, meaning that no abnormal cells have been detected.

Unsatisfactory. The cytologist did not have a good enough view to give a report, and the Pap should be repeated, usually in six to twelve weeks.

Inflammatory. May need treatment such as antibiotics for infection, and a repeat of the Pap test.

Atypia/LGSIL/ASCUS mild dysplasia/CIN 1. This reading means mild changes only, which may revert to normal. A small number of cells, if left untreated, may progress slowly to become a more severe problem and eventually to a cancer.

HGSIL/severe dysplasia/CIN 2 or 3. If you get this reading, it means severe changes, which need investigation and probably some treatment to prevent progress to cancer.

Cells typical of cervical cancer—a reading that rarely occurs. When it does occur, you should get treatment immediately.

Another way of expressing the same things is to term CIN 1 a "low-grade lesion" or LGSIL ("low-grade squamous intra-epithelial lesion"—what a mouthful!) and to lumping CIN 2 and CIN 3 together as "high-grade lesions" or HGSIL ("high-grade squamous intra-epithelial lesion"). All cytotechnicians and doctors who are involved in women's health recognize this terminology, known as the Bethesda classification, worldwide.

An older, but still easily recognizable terminology, is to speak in terms of "dysplasia" instead of CIN. In conversation, doctors still commonly use this term and modify it with "mild" meaning CIN 1 and "moderate" and "severe" denoting CIN 2 and CIN 3 respectively.

Sometimes, there are cells that are just not quite normal, but the changes aren't marked enough to merit being called CIN or dysplasia. In these cases, the cells are called "atypical"—or just not quite right. Very commonly, this is reported as ASCUS or "atypical squamous cells of uncertain significance," which is also part of the Bethesda classification. On a first reading of all these terms, they probably seem confusing, but when you work with them every day, the system is really quite simple.

The wart virus can also leave its telltale "fingerprint" on the cells of a Pap smear. When technicians recognize this, they will report the likely presence of HPV, human papilloma virus. This may be the first clue that HPV is present. We talk more about this virus and its significance later in the chapter.

Sometimes, a Pap smear may be reported out as "unsatisfactory." There are a number of common reasons for this: the slide may be obscured by too much blood (if you just had or are having your period); there may be signs of infection; not enough cells were obtained; the cells from the junction between the inner and outer skin of the cervix are not present; the cells may have gotten dried out and look like crunchy chips under the microscope; or there even may have been a broken slide. Any one of these is reason enough to repeat the Pap smear, after remedying whatever was the likely cause. If this happens to you, don't be upset with your doctor: it's just one of those things.

How often should you have a Pap test? Interval recommendations vary a bit with different countries. In the United States, the recommended interval for conventional Pap smears spread with a brush on a slide is every three years, after a woman has had three consecutive normal Pap smears, done at yearly intervals. Where ThinPrep with liquid-based cytology is used, the American Cancer Society recommends testing every two years until age thirty (provided reports are always negative). Thereafter, testing every three years is sufficient. Obviously recommendations differ for women who have been investigated or treated for abnormalities of the cervix. Women with high-risk HPV are screened annually. In Australia, Pap smears are recommended every two years; in the United Kingdom, the recommendation is every three years. Of course, no matter where you live the recommendation should be customized to your particular circumstances and your doctor is the one with whom to discuss this. It is also important to note that in countries like the United States, Australia, and the United Kingdom, at least half of the cervical cancer cases diagnosed are in women who have *never* had a Pap smear or who have not had one in more than five years. So, get your Pap smear!

A Pap smear is a screening test, and it's important for you to understand the implications and limitations of this fact. A screening test is an efficient, safe, relatively inexpensive way to test *large populations* for indicators of possible illness; in this case, women for possible signs of cervical precancer. A screening test is not 100 percent accurate and this applies to Pap smears, too. In fact, an inaccuracy rate of about 5 percent is considered acceptable for screening tests. The aim of a Pap test is to identify cells that may be precancerous or cancerous, then go on to investigate further, and treat what is found. The accuracy of a single Pap smear depends on many variables, but a series of Pap smears, done according to recommended intervals, greatly increases the probability of diagnosing a potential problem and instituting treatment at early stages.

In March 2003, the U.S. Food and Drug Administration (FDA) approved human papilloma virus (HPV) virus screening as an adjunct to the Pap test. HPV, also known as wart virus, is commonly found in the vaginal and cervical skin, most often in young women soon after they begin having sexual intercourse. Although some may experience warts, the vast majority does not have warts in the vagina or on the cervix. Most of their male partners do not have warts either—it is more common to have the wart virus present in the body without warts ever appearing than it is to have visible warts. There are over one hundred different strains of HPV, of which about twenty can be present on the cervix; and of these twenty, only a small number are associated with abnormal Pap reports and ultimately with the development of cervical cancer. These are referred to as "high-risk" HPV types and include types 16, 18, 31, 33, 35, 39, 45, 51, 52, 56, and 58. Most women whose Pap tests report HPV have low-risk types, usually 6, 11, 42, 43, or 44; moreover, in most women the normal mechanisms that combat infection in the body swing into action and deal with the HPV so that later Pap reports are normal. We also know that HPV is not the only factor responsible for causing cervical cancer; there are others that haven't been identified. (It's worth noting here that cigarette smoking increases your risk of cervical cancer, should you need yet another reason to give up the habit.)

Deaths from cervical cancer have dropped to a small fraction of what they were prior to the institution of routine Pap smear screening. We can thank the pioneering work of Dr. George Papanicolau for the introduction of Pap screening. Affectionately called "Dr. Pap," he began his medical career in his native Greece, where he met and married Andromache Mavroyenous, who became his helpmate in research as well as in life. The young couple immigrated to the United States after the Balkan War in 1912, and George soon began work at Cornell University, researching sex differentiation. It was while he was conducting research on guinea pigs that he noted that the vaginal secretions could give him valuable clues to the timing of ovulation. Mary, as Andromache was known in the United States, was his volunteer research assistant, and became a willing donor of vaginal specimens, as well. After examining vaginal secretions, Dr. Pap noted the secretions also yielded cancerous cells that might have application for detecting cancers in humans. This led to the development of the Pap smear and a revolution in preventive care for women, dramatically cutting the death rate from cervical cancer. Like many advances in medicine, recognition came slowly. Although Dr. Pap's and Mary's research with a group of women volunteers began in 1925, the value of the Pap smear and the use of vaginal and cervical cell studies wasn't recognized until the 1940s and not fully implemented in screening women for cervical cancer until the 1950s. And, of course, the recognition due to Andromache Papanicolau never came; today she undoubtedly would be recognized as a partner in achieving this medical advance.

Our fictitious character Dr. Hatch routinely uses a ThinPrep Pap. One reason she prefers this is that a DNA test for the HPV can be ordered easily using the same specimen. Remember, high-risk types of this virus are strongly correlated with cervical cancer and precancerous changes. She can do this two ways: simply by letting the lab know that she wants a high-risk HPV screen done, or that she wants this screen reflexively done if any abnormalities are noted or observed on the Pap smear. Because Frannie recently had unprotected sex, Dr. Hatch requested the HPV screen along with the Pap. A woman with a normal Pap smear and a negative HPV screen has only a 0.2 percent chance of later developing cervical cancer.

A separate test can be done for HPV either by using the Thin-Prep without a Pap or by using a different swab collection for HPV only. Both accomplish the same result; the choice depends on the lab your doctor uses. At present, HPV typing is not done routinely with a Pap smear, and whether or not it should be is still a topic of research and discussion. For women who have mild changes reported on their Paps tests (CIN 1) especially on several occasions, for older women, and for women with obvious warts, HPV typing may be very useful in either reassuring a woman and her doctor that she has a low-risk type, or in alerting them that she does have one of the high-risk types and therefore requires special attention and care.

The cytology lab that Dr. Hatch uses also routinely checks the smears it processes by computer. This has become increasingly common in the United States, but is by no means done by all labs. Two methods are in use: the one used by Dr. Hatch's lab, called Papnet, which looks twice at all smears; and the other, AutoPap, which looks again at all smears reported as normal. If you want to know which technology the lab used by your doctor employs, just ask your doctor. You have a right to know. (Keep in mind, however, that even with the best technology a small percentage of false positives and negatives still occur.) The lab Dr. Hatch uses also regularly provides education and feedback for doctors and nurses who take Pap smears.

False Positives

A false positive Pap smear suggests that a woman has some kind of precancerous cell changes when later diagnostic tests show she does not. Usually this happens because there is some infection or inflammation of the cervix. The report may read "possible high-grade lesion." In this situation it is common for a woman to have a colposcopy and biopsy (described in chapter 4). This is not a comfortable procedure and will cause a certain amount of psychological stress. However, once it is established that no serious problem exists, the woman can be reassured. It is also reassuring that there are no worrying side effects from the investigations. In our experience, most women realize that "it's better to be safe than sorry." It is also possible, as we've explained, that mild changes, particularly ASCUS and CIN 1, can resolve on their own, so even though the original Pap smear was reported correctly, by the time a colposcopy and biopsy are carried out the report shows completely normal results.

False Negatives

A false negative Pap smear may occur because not enough of the abnormal cells were picked up when the smear was taken, or because the technician failed to detect abnormal cells that were present. As we've described there are many checks in place to prevent false negatives from occurring. Nevertheless, some do slip through and this is one of the main reasons for recommending *regular* Paps. If you have a false negative on one occasion, it certainly should be detected the next time.

Why Aren't Pap Smears Always 100 Percent Right?

- Blood, mucus, or infections may prevent the cells from being picked up or make them difficult to see under the microscope.
- The right part of the cervix (what is called the squamo-columnar junction, where the skin outside of the cervix meets the lining tissue) may be difficult to reach—there may be scar tissue from previous births or surgeries. After menopause this junction is sometimes high inside the canal of the cervix.
- The spatula or brush doesn't touch the whole area and misses abnormal cells.
- The cells don't stick to the spatula or brush—this may happen particularly when a smear is taken during pregnancy.
- The smear is too thin or too thick.
- Only a few abnormal cells are present.
- The cytologist fails to detect an abnormality—cytologists are human too!

There are safeguards to try to prevent false negatives—making sure both types of cells are present, assessing smear quality, and checking with automated devices. Having regular smears is also a safeguard.

Other Cervical Screening Methods

In some parts of the world, universal Pap smear screening is prohibitively expensive and other methods are used. While generally recognized as less than ideal, they offer good compromise solutions in some areas of the third world.

When acetic acid (basically vinegar) is painted on the cervix, any abnormal cells turn white. Although often used in conjunction with our more technically sophisticated techniques (see chapter 4 on colposcopy), it is also used in underdeveloped areas as a means to identify places on the cervix from which biopsies or pieces of tissue are taken for pathologic examination. Nurses and midwives are trained to do this simple, cost-effective procedure that also has been found to be a reasonable screen for these populations. Another technique tried in certain remote communities is cervicography, in which a highly magnified photograph of the cervix is taken and later inspected by a doctor skilled at diagnosing abnormalities. Overall, however, Pap smears taken by hand and examined by qualified cytotechnologists have produced the best results.

We in the developed world are very fortunate to have cervical screening programs and access to the most advanced technologies. These screenings are not cost prohibitive for most women, and programs exist to aid those women whose access might be inhibited by cost. If you have any questions about access to any of these programs, just phone your local hospital, your state's health department, or Planned Parenthood.

Resources

INTERNET

Several websites listed in chapter 1 also contain information about Pap smear testing:

- *www.cancer.org*—the website of the American Cancer Society
- *www.cancernet.nci.nih.gov*—the information site of the National Cancer Institute
- *www.obgyn.net*—designed to provide information for the public

BOOKS

Buckman, Robert, and others. *What You Really Need to Know about Cancer.* Baltimore: Johns Hopkins University Press, 1997.

The Official Patients' Sourcebook on Cervical Cancer: A Revised and Updated Directory for the Internet Age. San Diego, Calif.: Icon Health Publications, 2002.

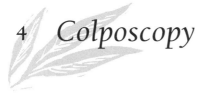

4 Colposcopy

Colposcopy is not, strictly speaking, a screening test because it is recommended only for women who have had an abnormal Pap smear report, rather than for the whole population of women. It is appropriate to include it here because it is an increasingly common procedure that women deserve to know more about. Colposcopy allows us to follow up abnormal Pap smears and do highly directed treatments and diagnostic biopsies on the cervix, as well as the vulva and vagina.

Returning to Frannie's case, she had a Pap smear done at her physical exam, and the results came back showing CIN 1, or LGSIL, a low-grade lesion indicative of HPV infection. HPV testing revealed HPV 11, a "low-risk" type. Frannie's friend and co-worker Brett also had a positive Pap smear; her HPV test showed 16, a "high-risk" type. Both women were scheduled to have a colposcopy done to help with diagnosis as well as treatment of the problem.

Frannie chose to go through a public hospital clinic; Brett did an Internet search to try to find the area's absolutely best gynecologist.

From this point on, both women had similar experiences and outcomes. Both had a colposcopy, the procedure now routinely done on any woman with more than a minor degree of abnormality on her Pap smear. The aim of colposcopy is to identify precancerous changes, to decide which are mild and likely to resolve themselves without treatment, and to treat those that are more serious, both to save life and to conserve future reproductive capabilities.

A colposcope is basically a magnifying telescope designed for looking at the skin of the cervix, and sometimes the vagina and vulva. There are changes characteristic of precancerous and cancerous lesions that can be seen on the surface of the cervix and in the blood vessels supplying it, changes that are more clearly visible when they are magnified by the colposcope. The examining doctor applies low-strength acetic acid—yep, vinegar—on the skin. Diseased areas show up against the healthy background because abnormal cells soak up more acetic acid than normal ones; they then stand out white against the nice healthy pink cells. Blood vessels show up better under a green light, and most colposcopes have both green and ordinary white light with which to view your cervix. A range of magnifications is also available.

Of course, in order for a doctor to see your cervix, you must have the speculum we've already described in your vagina. In the case of colposcopy, the speculum needs to be in place longer than it is for a simple Pap exam. This, of course, is not comfortable, but it should not be painful. (You can hedge your bets by taking a dose of ibuprofen prior to the exam.) You may be aware of a dripping sensation, of coldness from the vinegar, or a bit of a sting, but usually not more than this.

Your doctor usually has a nurse assisting who tells you what is expected from you at various points and can explain what the doctor is doing at any given moment. But more importantly, she gives you moral support and holds your hand if you feel a bit shaky. Alternatively, you can bring a friend or relative. Brett's best friend went along and was going to take Brett out for lunch after, even though Brett said, "I'm not sure I can go anywhere; I smell like a Caesar salad!"

Gynecologists usually perform colposcopies, although sometimes family doctors or nurse practitioners that have specialized training may do them. This is important because colposcopy, like Pap smear interpretation, depends entirely on the training and experience of the person performing the examination. The purpose of a colposcopy is to look at the relevant part of the cervix—what we call the "transformation zone." This is where the type of cell covering the outer portion of the cervix changes to that of the inner part of the cervical canal. It is at this place of meeting that most cancers begin. The doctor examines this area very carefully and takes biopsies of any areas that appear abnormal. These biopsies (sometimes one, sometimes more are taken) are tiny samples of suspicious tissue taken with special biopsy forceps—sort of like little pincers. We would be lying if we said that this was entirely pain free; the pain is momentary, rather like being bitten by a large mosquito, and again, taking ibuprofen helps. Bleeding occurs with the biopsy, but silver nitrate applicators or Monsell's paste may be used to stop it: these treatments are *not* painful.

After the colposcopy and biopsy, you can expect to have a bloody discharge for up to twenty-four hours; use pads or tampons that you change frequently and avoid vaginal intercourse until the discharge stops, allowing your tender cervix to heal.

Frannie felt faint and woozy after her biopsy, as some women do. Think of it as a quick bite taken from the cervix. Local anesthetic usually is not used, the argument being that instilling a local anesthetic actually hurts more than the quick snip with biopsy forceps. (Some doctors do use local anesthetic, like Novocain, and we don't quibble with that. They should tell you what they're doing as they go.) The nurse will tell you to take your time getting up and dressing. (Frannie felt quite okay after lying flat for a few minutes and drinking a glass of water.) Your doctor may discuss with you what she saw on your cervix, or she may wait until she also can discuss the lab report on the biopsy specimens. Even though you are not drugged, you may find the experience emotionally traumatizing enough that you don't remember what the doctor tells you at that time. Although doctors don't regard this as a major procedure, it looms much

larger for the woman who has experienced little of the technology we routinely employ. Go home, rest, and tell your family
that you are feeling a bit fragile and need them to be especially
caring.

Sometimes, especially after menopause, the junction between
the two types of cells may move far up into the cervix—too far
to see, even with the colposcope. This is a normal effect of the
reduced estrogen levels after menopause and no cause for alarm.
Your doctor may prescribe some topical estrogen cream to use
in the vagina and have you return for another try, or she may decide that it would be more appropriate to go on and do a surgical procedure to treat a presumptive area of abnormality.

If the cell changes are very mild, there may be nothing to
see on a colposcopy and you will be advised to have a repeat
Pap smear in three to six months, and sometimes, another colposcopy. In some cases, the changes seen by the doctor are exactly as predicted by your Pap smear; in others, they are more or
less serious than the Pap predicted. This is why we take biopsies:
a pathologist can examine the tissue under a microscope and
make a very accurate diagnosis. Of course, accuracy is dependent
upon your doctor's obtaining adequate biopsies from the correct
spots on your cervix. Again, this is a good reason to be sure your
doctor has enough experience doing this.

If your biopsy shows CIN 1, LGSIL, or mild dysplasia and this
is in agreement with your Pap and the visual findings on the colposcopy, then in all likelihood you will be told that no immediate treatment is necessary, but that you need to have another Pap
smear in three to six months. Don't think that you are being ne-
glected; lesions at this stage often go away completely on their
own, and follow-up tells us whether or not the problem is persistent and whether it is time to begin more aggressive treatment.

If the biopsy shows CIN 2 or 3 (also known as moderate or
severe dysplasia) or HGSIL, we suggest having treatment very
soon, so that the condition does not proceed to cancer. After all,
the idea behind all these tests is that no woman should go on to

have full-blown cervical cancer. We say to have treatment soon, meaning this is not an emergency; and if a woman receives this diagnosis during pregnancy, usually treatment usually is deferred until after the baby is delivered. That does not mean that you can ignore it for a few years and expect it to remain quiescent. Have treatment at your earliest convenience is probably the best way to express *soon*.

A biopsy seldom picks up full-blown cancer, but when it does treatment proceeds more urgently and is more extensive.

Frannie's biopsy showed CIN 1, which was consistent with her Pap and colposcopic findings. Her HPV test was positive but not for the high-risk strains of the virus. Four months later, her Pap smear and colposcopy were again normal. Frannie was immensely relieved, and she resolved never to have unprotected sex again.

Brett's biopsy was more serious, showing CIN 3, so Brett had laser treatment on her cervix. Although she, too, was sobered by these findings, her dominant emotions were of relief and gratitude at having had her Pap smear, which may have saved her life.

We hope that this demystifies having a colposcopy and demotes an abnormal Pap smear from a death notice to its rightful place as a first warning signal. These tests enable us to diagnose and cure lesions before they truly become cancer.

5 Screening for Breast Cancer

Jean Morris has been having mammograms since she was in her early forties. She doesn't really worry about breast cancer, as there is none in her family, but she knows it is smart to just go routinely and have her clinical breast exam and mammogram each year. "Now, Frannie, when you hit forty, you should start this, too. You'll hear all the jokes about how it feels—like lying on a concrete floor and having someone drive over your breasts or slamming the refrigerator door on them! But those are only jokes. Sure, it squeezes some, but it only lasts a few seconds and then it is done. Undetected breast cancer is a lot worse to deal with and lasts a lot longer."

Like many of us, Jean had lost a friend to breast cancer. Her best high school friend, Kathleen, developed breast cancer in her early forties and lost her battle in three short years. Kathleen had not had a screening mammogram because she thought she would wait another year or two. By then, she had found a lump the size of a small grape. Like many women, a combination of fear and optimism kept her from seeing the doctor immediately and the lump grew. The great irony was that Kathleen was a nurse who taught classes on women's health issues. Jean makes sure that her sister Bev and sister-in-law Rachel have regular mammograms, too; in fact, the last few years the women have made a day of it, all parading around together in their hospital gowns and having lunch at a nearby Italian place afterward.

Breast cancer is a disease in which cells of the breast tissue become malignant and invade other cells of the breast. It can spread to the lymph nodes and other organs, including the bones, brain, and liver. It is the second most commonly diagnosed cancer in women and the second leading cause of cancer death in women. Only skin cancer is more commonly diagnosed, and only lung cancer causes more deaths. In numbers, this means about 180,000 new cases of breast cancer are diagnosed annually in the United States. About 48,000 deaths occur every year. Obviously, prevention and early detection are the keys to reducing these numbers.

The risk factors for breast cancer include:

- Age. Forty is an important birthday to remember. Breast cancer is rare in women in their twenties and thirties except when there is a strong family history, but it becomes increasingly common with age.
- A first-degree relative with breast cancer that occurred premenopausally.
- A personal history of breast cancer or other premalignant breast disease.
- Hormone use.
- Caucasian race. This statement may be slightly misleading. Although African American women overall do have a slightly lower incidence of breast cancer than white women, they are more likely both to develop breast cancer before age fifty and to die from the condition.
- Radiation to the breasts or chest.
- Alcohol abuse.
- Early menarche (first period).
- Late first childbirth or no children.

A woman with several of these risk factors may want to discuss with her doctor the advisability of having a baseline mammogram before age forty.

Although we talk quite extensively about the high-tech tools used in screening for breast cancer, we must also emphasize the value of having a clinical breast exam every year. In administering this exam, a trained health professional looks at your breasts for any changes in skin texture or changes in symmetry and feels them for any lumps that should not be there. This is one of the reasons that women are encouraged to have a well-woman exam each year; it's also what makes this exam relevant for everyone—even the woman who has had a hysterectomy and has no health problems that she can identify. It doesn't all happen below the waist!

The breast self-exam (BSE) is another important topic. BSE has long been a part of the teaching provided to women by organizations such as the American Cancer Society, Planned Parenthood, and a multitude of women's self-help groups. Recently, evidence-based medicine proponents have raised questions about the value of this exercise. One argument is that a clinical exam and mammography detect breast cancers before they are palpable to the average woman. While we have no intention of arguing the issue, we do believe that there is no harm in examining your breasts each month (they are yours, after all). And, by the way, both of us have known women who found their breast cancers. Knowing your own body cannot be a bad thing.

When examining your breasts, first observe them from a full frontal view. Make sure that they are symmetrical and that you don't see skin changes, such as dimpling on the breast or skin that resembles that of an orange. Next, lean forward and make sure your breasts hang freely and symmetrically. Many women have breasts that differ slightly from each other in size and shape, and that is normal. Some asymmetry is to be expected, provided there has been no change since the last exam.

Next, raise one arm over your head, to stretch and flatten the muscles underlying the breast on that side. Then, with the flats of your fingers, feel your breast. There are two basic methods of doing this; pick one and become familiar with your own breasts.

The first, illustrated in most American Cancer Society booklets, is concentric circles. Using this method, you start at the areola and move around the breast, feeling with the flats of your fingers and keep going around in concentric circles until you have felt the entire breast. The other method, which we learned in medical school in Ireland, is like sectioning wedges of a pie. You start in the muscle line at the front of the armpit and feel with the flats of your fingers in toward the nipple, moving in this way from segment to segment until you complete the full circle and are back where you began. There is no real reason to advocate one method over the other, as long as you are methodical and feel all the breast tissue.

It is a good idea to first examine your breasts on the same day that you have had a professional exam; this way you know that what you are feeling is normal. Each woman's breasts feel a little bit different from others, and it is important to know the normal feel of your own breasts. If you are still menstruating, it is also a good idea to examine your breasts only in the week after your period, because that is when they are least lumpy.

If you find something in your breast that seems abnormal for you, do not immediately assume the worst. Small cysts (collections of fluid) are common in the breasts of young women, and are harmless. Also, do not be so frightened by it that you try to ignore it. Go see your doctor and have a professional exam. Perhaps a mammogram or ultrasound will be ordered (see later in this chapter), perhaps the opinion of a surgeon will be sought, but remember that 85 percent of the masses found in breasts are benign or noncancerous. The odds of your finding breast cancer are small, but it is vital that you check it out.

A mammogram is suggested for every woman in the United States from age forty on. Although there is some debate about the cost-benefit relationship of annual mammograms for women in the forty-to-fifty age group, the American Cancer Society and National Cancer Institute still recommend them because the benefit to the individual identified as having breast cancer is irrefutable. In Australia, the recommended interval for this age group is two years. (There's also some discussion about the implications of false positives, which we'll refer to shortly.)

A mammogram is an X-ray of the breast using special X-ray equipment. You can feel secure that this equipment exposes you to very little radiation and that having mammograms according to current guidelines does not increase your risk of cancer caused by radiation. This has been thoroughly studied.

We recommend using a facility that does many mammograms, so that you have the benefit of highly experienced radiologists. Once you are happy with a mammography facility, it's best to keep using it so they can compare your mammograms from year to year. If you move and have to change facilities, ask for your old films to be transferred, not just the written reports. Jean, Bev, and Rachel all go to the local breast center where they are "old hands." Like all mammography facilities in the United States, it is certified by the appropriate credentialing bodies, which means every mammogram machine used within it is approved by the FDA.

When you arrive at the mammography suite in the outpatient section of a hospital or at a freestanding breast center, you are shown to a cubicle where you remove all your clothes, including jewelry, from the waist up. Remember to wear a shirt or blouse with a skirt or trousers, so you only need to strip down to your waist. It is best to avoid wearing deodorant or body powder that day because these can cause puzzling shadows on the X-ray that inhibit accurate reading. You put on a hospital gown and leave it open in the front. (As Jean said, "No fashion statements here.")

The X-ray technician, who is especially trained and certified in doing mammograms, is usually a woman. She takes you into the mammography room and positions you standing against the X-ray machine. Your arm is angled back out of the way in order to position your breast against a film cassette. When in place, the breast is compressed by a plastic paddle. She does each breast separately, repositioning and compressing each breast twice to take photos in both a horizontal and vertical direction. Compression thins out the breast tissue to get a good view all through it. (You might imagine your breast as pancake mixture, spreading it out so that it cooks evenly.) It is not comfortable, but you stay in each position for only a matter of seconds and it rarely hurts. You are usually at the mammogram center for about thirty to forty-five minutes. If time is a limiting factor for you, try booking the first appointment of the day.

Women who have breast implants should make this fact known to their X-ray technician. Implants are usually inserted between the chest wall and the natural breast tissue, but sometimes they are placed under the muscle of the chest wall. In either case, the technician is able to identify the breast tissue appearances on the films, and knows to carefully avoid using too much pressure, which might rupture the implants. Sometimes several more lateral views are needed for women with implants because the silicone in implants does not allow X-rays of the mammogram to pass through. It should be possible to view all the natural breast tissue of women who have implants.

All health insurance in the United States now covers mammography. It is more cost effective to detect and treat an early breast cancer than it is to delay diagnosis. For women who do not have coverage, most, if not all states have special programs to cover screening mammograms for women age fifty and older, as well as for younger women at high risk. These plans do have an income eligibility screen. Many community hospitals and breast centers offer mammograms either free or at deeply reduced rates during Breast Cancer Awareness Month. Call your local American Cancer Society office for information about these and other community programs that may be helpful.

It is important to understand the limitations of screening mammography. As we have said, screening tests are not diagnostic procedures, and each involves an acceptable level of false positives and negatives. This is the nature of screening. And having a mammogram does not *protect* a woman against breast cancer—like a Pap smear, it is designed to pick up early changes that if left alone may develop into widespread cancer.

We also need to distinguish between screening mammograms and diagnostic mammograms. Screening mammograms are the routine procedures done on a yearly basis that we've described for Jean, Bev, and Rachel. Diagnostic mammograms are done because a woman has a specific problem, such as a lump she or her doctor has found on examination, a discharge from one of her nipples, or because an abnormality has been found on a screening mammogram. A diagnostic mammogram involves taking more pictures than it does for a screening mammogram, and they will be concentrated on one or more areas of the breasts.

What do mammograms actually show? When you look at your films you see black-and-white images of your breasts. These are carefully inspected by a trained radiologist, a doctor who is Board-certified in his or her specialty, who then compares them with previous mammograms. It is not uncommon to see white deposits of calcium on mammograms. If these are relatively large (macrocalcification), they are age-related changes of no worrying significance. Smaller specks of calcium (microcalcification), however, may indicate suspicious areas. There also may be one or more lumps, or masses, of breast tissue, which to the trained radiologist's eye appears abnormal. Sometimes such a mass is simply a collection of fluid, a cyst, which is benign, and sometimes the mass is simply normal breast tissue. But, on occasion, such a mass may be a cancer. To make a more definite diagnosis, either the radiologist, a surgeon, or other doctor who is expert in breast care may recommend further mammograms and/or an ultrasound or biopsy.

Your mammogram should be reported in a standard way developed by the American College of Radiology. Called BI-RADS, it is comparable to the Pap smear reporting system we've already described. Breast Imaging and Reporting and Data System, or BI-RADS, uses the following ratings:

- Category 0—a complete report cannot be given because complete views of the breast were not obtained, or further tests such as breast ultrasound are recommended.
- Category 1—negative. Good news! Both breasts appear completely normal.
- Category 2—benign findings. This means some change has been noted but that change is benign (noncancerous). It's important to have such changes noted so they are not misinterpreted in future mammograms.
- Category 3—probably benign findings. This means just what it says. The usual practice is to repeat the mammogram, perhaps in six months, to see if an area is changing. (Please note that breast cancer develops *slowly*.) This avoids unnecessary biopsies, but makes sure that if the area is becoming abnormal action is taken in time.
- Category 4—suspicious findings. Biopsy recommended.
- Category 5—highly suggestive of breast cancer. Action should be taken ASAP.

Fortunately, Jean, Bev, and Rachel have had negative mammogram results so far.

What rate of false results can be expected? In women between the ages of forty and sixty-nine in the United States, there is a 30 percent chance of receiving a false positive over a ten-year period. This is about twice the rate of false positives in Great Britain and some European countries and is the subject of ongoing discussion among breast cancer experts in the United States. (In the United States, mammography screening starts at age forty; as a rule, it is not yearly between the ages of forty and fifty, but women over fifty are screened every year. In Great Britain screening is only every two years. Despite this, the rates of breast cancer detection are very similar in the two countries.)

These false positives have a high cost in terms of emotional distress as well as the costs and stress of additional testing. Biopsies and surgeries to remove lumps may be done, ultimately proving that it has been a false alarm. On the other end of the spectrum, 10 to 15 percent of all breast cancers may not be detected by a single mammogram. Despite these figures, most doctors involved in the detection and treatment of breast cancer, as well as the American Cancer Society, the National Cancer Institute, and the American College of Surgeons, currently believe it is worth having routine screening mammograms and clinical breast exams because they continue to be our best defense against breast cancer mortality. Any woman who has a life expectancy of more than five years should continue to have routine mammograms. Breast cancer is more common as we grow older, and many older women with breast cancer die from unrelated illnesses. Of course, you have the right to be well informed about all the positive and negative aspects of mammograms before deciding whether or not to have one.

One area of controversy concerns the condition of ductal carcinoma-in-situ (DCIS). In this condition abnormal cells are found in the breast tissue, but are confined to the milk ducts (narrow passages within the breast, leading to the nipple). This is somewhat like the CIN 3 that may be found on Pap smears. DCIS is most often picked up initially by mammogram, rather than by a woman feeling a lump or noticing a discharge from her nipple. Doctors now realize that although DCIS can and does often progress to frank, invasive cancer, it does not always do so. In the past some women have had mastectomies for DCIS as protective measures against cancer, when it is possible that they may never have developed cancer. On the other hand, many women undoubtedly have been saved from progressive cancer by such treatment. Now breast physicians and surgeons realize that in some women treatment less radical than mastectomy may be adequate for DCIS. Detailed discussion of the diagnosis of breast cancer and explanations about treatments are beyond the scope of this book, but other sources of information are listed in reference sections. What concerns us is that this controversy has been used by some people to argue against having mammograms at all—a classic case of shooting the messenger, rather than taking note of the message, we believe. DCIS is most often found after microcalcification is seen on a mammogram. If this happens to you, expect to have further investigation and detailed discussion with a doctor who is an expert in breast disease. You can then make up your mind what course to follow. It seems far better to us to have the mammogram and then act on any implications of the results, rather than to decide not to have it because there's a tiny chance that you might end up having more surgery than necessary. Yes, occasionally a woman has surgery based on a mammogram that is possibly more extensive than needed. Balance this information against the fact that breast exams and mammograms are the most effective methods of screening for early breast cancer—and they are very effective—and we think you'll agree with us and all the relevant expert bodies that having these tests at the recommended intervals is a sensible thing to do.

Tools that help improve the accuracy of breast cancer detection are ultrasound, digital mammography, and breast MRI. And, of course, biopsies add further clarity if abnormalities are found with these imaging methods.

An ultrasound is produced by passing high-frequency sound waves through tissue, in this case, breast tissue. Like radar, the waves bounce off different surfaces within the tissue, and the returning waves are converted into picture form on the ultrasound screen. Ultrasound tests are done on an outpatient basis, frequently in the same suite as the mammogram. Today, it is not uncommon for a mammogram to be followed by an ultrasound of one or both breasts at the radiologist's recommendation. An ultrasound can help differentiate between solid and cystic masses in the breast, especially when a palpable mass has been found on clinical breast exam and is not well visualized by mammogram. It is also very helpful in younger women who naturally tend to have denser breast tissue; it is safe, takes about as long as a mammogram, and does not hurt. Like mammograms, women technicians usually do the breast ultrasound. Ultrasound, alone, is not an adequate screen for breast cancer. It is only useful as an adjunct to mammography.

Digital mammography is not yet routinely used, but may offer some advantages over conventional mammography in that the images can be stored digitally and the brightness or contrast can be manipulated to allow better visualization. Eventually, it also may be used to transmit mammograms across telephone or wireless channels for interpretation or consultation at a distance, which would be useful for rural centers. Computerized analysis may also come into play, although these uses are not yet FDA approved.

Breast MRI is coming into its own, moving out of academic research centers and into community hospital use. Some experts suggest that it offers 95 percent accuracy in detecting breast cancers. An MRI is a procedure in which images produced by exposing the breast to a powerful electromagnetic field are analyzed by a computer. For a breast MRI, you lie face down, with your arms up and your head supported by your arms and pillows. Your breasts are placed in special breast MRI coils (these are the electromagnet) and a contrast agent is administered intravenously.

Breast MRI is an adjunct to routine mammography and clinical breast exam. Indications for a breast MRI are:

- Women with first-degree relatives with breast cancer, or women with the breast cancer genetic trait (discussed later in this chapter).
- Women with a suspicious or ambiguous mammography finding, as recommended by the radiologist.

- Preoperative diagnostic MRI for women who have had a positive biopsy, either by fine-needle aspiration or by a core biopsy.
- Follow-up MRI six months after an excisional biopsy for breast cancer, that is, if the biopsy removed the whole abnormal area, if an MRI was not previously done.
- Women who have a history of breast cancer or precancerous breast disease (although for women in this category who have had chemotherapy MRI may be less accurate).

Considerations and contraindications:

- An MRI is contraindicated in anyone who has bits of metal in their bodies; examples of this are pacemakers, angio clips, staples from previous surgery, or various implants.
- Hormonal replacement must be stopped for at least six weeks prior to breast MRI. Hormones make the breasts more dense and more difficult to image.
- For technical reasons, a woman cannot weigh more than 250 pounds. It is not intended to be a discriminatory or limiting factor.
- Premenopausal women must be scheduled for MRIs within one week after the menses.
- Breast cancer patients must wait six months after completing radiation treatments before having a breast MRI.
- A claustrophobic person may require premedication.

Again, we must reiterate that at this time, the breast MRI is a diagnostic test used in the circumstances described and is not a screening test.

A breast biopsy is not a screening test, but is a follow-up diagnostic test done when a clinical exam or mammography indicates a suspicious lesion. A biopsy is a surgically obtained specimen of breast tissue that is examined under the microscope by a pathologist. Biopsies can be done three separate ways:

- A fine-needle aspiration is done with a very fine needle directed by ultrasound, or stereotactic technique (sort of like robotics), to the right area in the breast. Once there, a tiny amount of tissue is sucked up through the needle and sent to the laboratory for examination by the pathologist.
- A core-needle biopsy uses a larger needle to obtain a core of tissue, in much the same manner as the fine-needle aspiration.
- Excisional biopsy may be done when there is a palpable mass; the mass is cut out and sent for pathology examination.

Local anesthetic, or in some cases general anesthesia, is used to numb the area before a breast biopsy. The type of anesthesia used depends on exactly what is being done, and should be clearly explained beforehand by your doctor.

Examination of tissue obtained from a breast biopsy is usually complete within a day or so, and you should then expect to discuss the findings and implications with your doctor. Waiting for an appointment for a breast biopsy, then waiting for the results— though usually only a matter of days—is not a happy time for any woman. Seek the help and support of partners, family, and friends, and try to keep other stresses to a minimum.

Breast biopsies may be done by surgeons or radiologists, or a combination of both. Doctors with a great deal of experience consistently produce the best results. Lists of accredited doctors and facilities can be obtained through the websites mentioned in the resources section at the end of the chapter. The implications of positive findings on breast biopsy are beyond the scope of our book; but you can find information through these websites and the resources in the Further Reading section.

Screening for Genetic Risk of Breast Cancer

Some families are unlucky. Women of Ashkenazi Jewish origin, for example, as well as those of a number of other ethnic groups, are at greater risk for genetically determined breast cancer. While about 10 to 15 percent of breast cancers in the general population are associated with familial risk factors, about one third of the cancers in these groups are associated with the so-called breast cancer genes. Known in the scientific community as BRCA 1 and BRCA 2, these genes occur in 1 percent of Ashkenazi Jewish women. In the general population, they are found in 0.12 percent of women. These genes are linked not only with breast cancer, but also with ovarian and colon cancer.

Screening for these genes is appropriate in women of Ashkenazi Jewish origin with a family history of breast cancer and in any woman with a strong family history of breast and/or ovarian cancer. We tell you more about this through the story of Kathleen's family, in whom the BRCA 1 gene was passed from mother to daughter, in chapter 15 on genetic testing. If any of these indications apply to you, discuss them at length with your doctor, including what steps to take if you are diagnosed as having one of these genes. The existing guidelines suggest early self-exam, yearly clinical breast exam, and annual mammography beginning at age twenty-five. Although some women with these genes opt for bilateral mastectomy as a prophylactic measure, there is insufficient evidence to suggest this course of action for everyone.

In the future, we may be puffing in a breath analyzer to do our breast cancer screen. Studies are showing that women with breast cancer have increased markers for oxidative stress in their breath that can be measured. Breath samples distinguish between healthy women and women with breast cancer at a sensitivity of 94.1 percent and a specificity (that is, breast cancer is truly causing the change) of 73.8 percent in studies done so far.

This technology is very promising and its development is being closely monitored.

Resources

INTERNET

In addition to much useful information on the American Cancer Society and National Cancer Institute websites, you can find all FDA-certified mammography sites at *www.fda.gov/cdrh/ mammography/certified.html*. The American College of Radiology website is *www.acr.org* and contains up-to-date information about accredited facilities, BI-RADS, and other topics accessible to lay readers. The website of the American College of Surgeons, *www.facs.org*, also provides some information for the general public as well as a list of publications. Also helpful are *www.aafp .org*, the website of the American Academy of Family Physicians, and *www.WebMD.com*, a reliable commercial site.

BOOKS

American Cancer Society. *A Breast Cancer Journey: Your Personal Guidebook*. 2d ed. Atlanta: ACS, 2004.

Love, Susan M., and Karen Lindsey. *Dr. Susan Love's Breast Book*. Boulder, CO: Perseus Publishing, 2000.

6 *Screening for Colon Cancer*

At the age of fifty-five, Jean Morris had a fright. One morning she found bright red blood on the toilet tissue. Her first thought was "those pesky hemorrhoids," but the next thought was of her mother, who died at sixty-seven of colon cancer. Like many people, Jean had been reluctant to listen to her doctor's advice about colon cancer screening. It was gross; it was embarrassing; she didn't have time for it. Millions of reasons—or excuses.

Katie Couric, of TV celebrity, has raised the consciousness of many Americans about colon cancer and the screening available to catch it early. Her husband died tragically young at age forty-two of colon cancer and her crusade against the disease serves as a memorial to him.

Cancer of the colon and rectum (sometimes called cancer of the bowel) is the third most common cancer in the United States. In the year 2000 alone, it caused an estimated 56,300 deaths. (These figures are for men and women combined.) It was estimated that about 180,000 new cases would be diagnosed in the United States in 2003. And these are just the U.S. statistics. Although treatment of this dreaded disease has improved, the best means of improving survival is still early detection . . . and this means screening for the unannounced presence of the disease.

There is some division among experts as to what is the best colon cancer screening protocol for the general public, but there is more unanimity in the recommendations for high-risk persons. Who is high risk? Any person who has a first-degree relative who has had colon cancer before the age of sixty; anyone who has had two or more first-degree relatives with colon cancer regardless of age; and any person who has a personal history of colon cancer, adenomatous polyps in the colon, or ulcerative colitis—all are at high risk. It is agreed that screening in this population should begin at an earlier age, usually at age forty, but if many family members have had the illness, screening may begin much earlier. For people at high risk, family history is extremely important. We refer to this in more detail in the chapter on genetic screening.

It is recommended that people who are part of this risk group have an annual fecal occult blood test (FOBT) and regular endoscopic examination. Usually this means a *colonoscopy* (examination of the entire bowel with a telescope), which is our recommendation for this group. We'll explain the how and what happens of these tests in a moment.

For people who do not fall into the high-risk category, the recommendations are unanimous that all people should be screened from age fifty on and that FOBT should be done annually. There is also the strongest evidence base for the FOBT test being a reasonable screen in the low-risk population. The American Cancer Society, American Gastroenterological Association, and the American Academy of Family Practice also recommend flexible *sigmoidoscopy* (also an examination of the lower bowel with a telescope) every five years and colonoscopy every ten years. Sometimes, a double-contrast barium enema, a kind of X-ray, is recommended in place of sigmoidoscopy or colonoscopy.

Because she had a show of blood and her mother had died of colon cancer, Jean is high risk. After explaining this to her, Dr. Most scheduled Jean for a colonoscopy. He explained that she would be lightly sedated, so that her muscles could relax but she could still be able to cooperate during the exam and that he would be using a fiber-optic instrument that could be thought of as a sort of high-tech garden hose to thread up through her rectum and the length of her large bowel.

"Oh great," said Jean, "sounds like just the way I'd like to spend my day off work!"

Dr. Most explained to Jean that it would be necessary for her to do a special preparation the day before the exam, so that her colon would be as clean as possible, since stool in the colon can obstruct vision and make the test a failure.

Jean was given printed instructions by Lisa, the office nurse. These advised her to:

1. Eat no solid foods for twenty-four hours prior to the exam and drink only clear liquids.
2. Avoid aspirin, iron, and NSAID drugs such as ibuprofen for five days prior to the exam.
3. Take the prescribed laxative with large quantities of water and clear liquids the day prior to the exam.

(Each doctor has a personal preference for particular laxative preps, so we'll leave that to your doctor. You should be aware that once in a while, even when instructions are carefully followed, the colon may not be adequately clean at the time of the procedure and further cleansing may be necessary. If this happens to you, don't feel embarrassed—we assure you that all technical procedures can have little glitches.)

Jean was instructed to be near a toilet the day before the exam, as the laxative would necessitate frequent visits. It was further explained that she should arrange for a companion to drive her home after the test as the sedative could make her drowsy. It didn't apply to Jean, but if you have a history of any valvular heart disease, your doctor will also give you an antibiotic before performing this exam. Lastly, Jean was instructed that when she arrived at the hospital, she would be asked to disrobe and change into a hospital gown and that she would next see Dr. Most in the exam room. Lisa reassured Jean that she would be present to answer all her questions and to hold her hand; in addition, she would be available to assist Dr. Most in the unlikely event of a problem's developing. Dr. Most does all his colono-scopies either in the outpatient unit of Jean's local hospital or in a free-standing certified facility designed for such procedures. It is important, if problems do arise, that equipment and staff are on hand to deal with them. (For a list of such facilities in your area, consult one of the websites we've already recommended.)

On the scheduled day, Jean arrived at the hospital and signed in. All she could think of was how she'd love a cup of coffee, but she would have to wait. She had used a small Fleet enema just after arising and was feeling a little desperate for the toilet.

Eventually, Jean was alone in a small room with Lisa and Dr. Most. Lisa had inserted an IV in the back of Jean's hand to ad-minister some sedation, so Jean was feeling very drowsy and far away. Jean had been questioned earlier about any drug allergies (she has none), as very rarely reactions can occur during the procedure to the medications used for sedation. Lisa helped Jean to position herself on the hospital bed, lying on her left side, with her right leg flexed and pulled up. It was nearly the same position in which Jean sleeps. On her right index finger, Lisa clipped a clothespin-like device, which she explained was a pulse oximeter that measured the oxygen level in Jean's blood. Dr. Most then asked Jean if she was ready to begin.

When Jean responded that she was ready, Dr. Most inserted his lubricated and gloved index finger into Jean's rectum and examined it for any obvious lumps or bumps. He then gently inserted the lubricated colonoscope, a hoselike fiber-optic in-strument about four feet long, into Jean's rectum and threaded it gently up along Jean's colon. Through the monitor attached to the colonoscope, Dr. Most was able to look at the entire length of Jean's colon; he showed her what it looked like and told her he'd shoot a few photos for her picture album. He explained that if Jean's bowel prep hadn't been as good as it was, he could have used a stream of water to clean certain areas, but was happy that wasn't necessary. At one point, Jean felt a little cramping discomfort and Dr. Most apologized; he'd just blown a little air into the colon to better enable him to see a particular spot.

"Look, Jean, see this little mushroomlike bit of flesh on the wall of your colon? That's a polyp and I'm going to remove it through the colonoscope and send it for biopsy. It may be the reason you bled, and I'll look to see if there are more. You'll also hear a sucking noise, as I suction a little pocket of liquid feces; don't worry—nothing's wrong."

Dr. Most carefully and methodically examined the whole length of Jean's colon and found two small polyps, both of which he removed through the colonoscope and sent for pathologic exam. He then carefully and gently removed the colonoscope, and Lisa removed the IV from Jean's hand and said, "We're just going to let you rest a bit before you try to jump up and go home, Jean. In a few minutes, I'll ask Frannie to come in and help you get dressed." Dr. Most also scheduled an appointment for Jean to come and discuss the findings and pathology results a few days later. Although you might expect your doctor to talk to you about your procedure at the time, the effects of the drugs used for sedation and the stress of the procedure itself can make it hard to take in much information—it's best discussed later when you are recovered and wide awake. Some colonoscopies are done with the assistance of an anesthesiologist; sedation is deeper and you certainly won't remember the procedure—all information should be discussed with you at least hours, if not days, later.

The preparation and procedure for a flexible sigmoidoscopy is virtually identical to that of the colonoscopy. The main difference between the two procedures is that the sigmoidoscope is only about twenty-five inches long and the doctor can only visualize the descending or left side of the colon. In a low-risk patient, this may be adequate.

Endoscopy (examination of the bowel with a colonoscope or sigmoidoscope) does have some risks you need to be aware of and discuss with your surgeon or gastroenterologist (a doctor specializing in diseases of the stomach and bowel) prior to consenting to your procedure. Rarely there may be a reaction to the drugs used for sedation, necessitating urgent treatment by your doctor; and in fact, the procedure may have to be abandoned until another day. Occasionally patients may vomit during the procedure; because of the sedation, it is important to have a trained nurse like Lisa on hand to prevent aspiration of vomit into the lungs. It is also possible for the telescope to perforate the wall of the colon or it may happen while a polyp is being cut off the inside of the bowel wall. In this situation, a larger surgery may be needed to repair the hole. Bleeding also may be caused by the endoscopy, which may need further surgery to control. You can ask your doctor beforehand about his or her rate of such complications—you would expect a figure of less than 1 percent. Most people feel that this small risk is justified by the peace of mind brought by learning that they don't have colon cancer; or if they do, that it has been detected early. However, you must be well informed before consenting to endoscopy.

Because of her grandmother's cancer and her mom's recent scare, Frannie decided that she'd start doing the FOBT yearly, even though she is still younger than most doctors start screening. "After all," she reasoned, "this test is so cheap and simple that I have nothing to lose. I can even afford to pay for it myself, if my insurance won't pay."

The fecal occult blood test is a simple one that detects minute amounts of blood in the stool. It is based on a simple chemical reaction of blood with a developing chemical, giving a distinctive blue color when blood is present. It is estimated that if everyone over age fifty did this simple test every year, the colon cancer death rate would be cut by 30 percent.

To most effectively use the fecal occult blood test, you should follow these simple directions for the three days before testing and during the three days that you collect stool samples:

- Don't take supplemental Vitamin C or eat large amounts of foods containing Vitamin C, such as citrus fruits.

- Do not eat red meat.
- Avoid or eat only small amounts of foods in the cabbage family.
- Avoid iron supplements, aspirin, and analgesics such as ibuprofen and naproxen. (You can take acetaminophen during the time period involved.)

You will be given three little stool cards and three "Popsicle sticks" with which to spread the stool on the paper in the stool card. There are several ways to collect stool samples:

1. Defecate into small plastic containers,
2. spread plastic wrap over the toilet bowl and after urinating into the toilet, defecate onto the plastic, or
3. if you are sure you have no bleeding hemorrhoid or little cut around the anus, dab at the stool as you defecate.

At the end of the day, any of these will get the job done. After you have collected the stool, spread a small dab of it on the little area indicated on the stool card; and, when you have three consecutive days' collection, either take or mail it back to your doctor. Some doctors have them sent to a lab; if your doctor prefers this, you'll be told where to send them. At the office or lab, a developing chemical is dropped on the stool card and if blood is present, the area will turn blue. All stool cards incorporate a control that turns blue with the chemical so that we know the test is not faulty. We ask for three consecutive days of samples because bowel lesions tend to bleed intermittently and this increases the probability of picking up a bleeding polyp, ulcer, or cancer. If the test is positive for blood, the patient is scheduled for a colonoscopy. (Remember: a screen is not diagnostic and when positive, simply indicates the need for more definitive tests.)

False positive results can occur because you've recently swallowed one of the substances we've listed. A false positive can also occur because you have some bleeding from a condition like a

*Colon Cancer Screening Recommendations
for Low-Risk Adults*

- Fecal occult blood test yearly from age fifty.
- Sigmoidoscopy every five years from age fifty.
- Colonoscopy every ten years from age fifty.
- Double-contrast barium enema may replace sigmoidoscopy/ colonoscopy in some persons.

polyp that nevertheless proves to be benign (not a cancer). So, a false positive may lead to your having a colonoscopy in order to show that you do not have cancer, and of course the colonoscopy carries the small but definite risks we've described. You also need to be aware of this: False negatives can occur because a genuine cancer was not bleeding at the time of testing. Regular testing and following the guidelines for colon cancer screening reduce the chances of a cancer's not being picked up.

Researchers are excited about a new fecal occult blood test, called !nSure. This test is done by swabbing the stool in the toilet water with a brush after a bowel movement, instead of using a wooden spatula to obtain samples from stool caught in a container. Probably because of this sampling method and the lack of need for dietary restrictions, it was found to be 74 percent more acceptable to the general public. !nSure does not require the dietary and drug restrictions of the card-based tests and has been demonstrated to be 85 percent sensitive for detecting cancer versus 39 percent for the card-based test. Both tests have a 4 percent false positive rate. !nSure requires only one sample of stool for testing. This test is based on specific chemicals that are present in blood and is more specific than the conventional fecal occult blood test.

Another breakthrough hovering on the horizon is a stool test that detects cancer DNA markers and promises to be the best non-invasive screen yet for colon cancer. It has recently become commercially available and should become widely available in the future. People find it more acceptable than traditional fecal occult blood tests because it is simple to use, requires the collection of one bowel movement, and doesn't require any dietary restrictions prior to doing the test. It is hoped that eventually this test will be a screening test that is diagnostic as well, although it is not currently recommended to replace colonoscopy in high-risk persons. The test is called PreGen-Plus.

When Jean's sister, Beverly, had a colonoscopy, her doctor was unable to visualize the entire colon for two reasons: Bev's bowel prep hadn't worked well enough and there was still a lot of stool obscuring the doctor's vision (too much to clean with a little spray and suction through the colonoscope); and maybe because of the retained stool difficulties, Beverly was cramping up too much and the procedure became technically difficult. Of course, Bev didn't remember a bit of this, thanks to the sedation, but her doctor phoned the next morning and discussed it with her. He suggested that she have a double-contrast barium enema, since it really was important to do as good a screen as possible, given her family history.

"Oh great, now I get to do that prep all over again!" Bev grumbled to her family. And, yes, the preparation for the double-contrast barium enema is like that for the endoscopic procedures: clear liquid diet and laxatives the day before and maybe an enema on the morning of the test. No fun, but necessary.

In the X-ray suite (or Medical Imaging Department, as it is often called), Bev put on a gown and "assumed the position" just as she had done for the attempted colonoscopy; only this time, she was given an enema of barium, which is a heavy white substance that blocks the penetration of X-rays and shows up as clearly delineated white areas on X-ray films. "Double-contrast" means that air was puffed into her rectum through the tube used for the enema, basically blowing the colon up a little bit like a balloon. This can be uncomfortable, but allows for better visualization of any abnormalities in the colon, especially smaller ulcers or

Table 6.1 Comparison of Colon Cancer Screens

Procedure	Cost	Advantage	Disadvantage	Risks
FOBT	$	Non-invasive	Nondiagnostic	None
Flexible sigmoidoscopy	$$	Can be done in office, biopsies can be done	Invasive, uncomfortable	Perforation 0.002% to 0.0001%, pain, bleeding, infection
Colonoscopy	$$$	Direct vision of whole colon, biopsies can be done	Invasive, uncomfortable, sedation required; expensive	Perforation 0.01% to 0.5%, bleeding, infection, dehydration
Double-contrast barium enema	$$	Less invasive than colonoscopy	Radiation exposure	Radiation exposure, bowel obstruction

polyps. X-ray pictures are taken. After the procedure, Beverly was given yet another laxative to take that evening to make sure that all the barium got cleaned out. Although she wasn't happy about going through these procedures, her peace of mind was definitely worth it. Oh yes, both Beverly and Jean were found to be free of cancer, and Frannie had no blood in her stool.

We're often asked what constitutes a clear liquid diet. Clear liquids are tea or coffee without milk or artificial creamers, strained juices, broth or bouillon, water, Jell-O, Popsicles, carbonated drinks, and sorbet or fruit ice. No dairy products or red-colored foods or drinks are allowed.

In the foreseeable future, virtual colonoscopy may become another screening tool. Virtual colonoscopy is an imaging test of the bowel using CT scan technology. Researchers have been looking at this as a non-invasive screen for bowel tumors for quite some time; but recently, researchers at several armed services hospitals found that utilizing a contrast medium (a dye that you swallow) to highlight tumors along with a three-dimensional approach to the CT viewing makes virtual colonoscopy much more sensitive. In fact, for larger lesions that are clinically more significant (that is, more likely to be cancerous), the virtual colonoscopy outperformed conventional colonoscopy. Still, virtual colonoscopy is not as good as conventional colonoscopy for identifying small lesions, nor can you remove a polyp or do a biopsy using virtual colonoscopy. For these purposes, a conventional colonoscopy is still the tool of choice.

Virtual colonoscopy is also expensive. It costs several thousand dollars and is not covered by most insurance plans yet. In the future, these roadblocks are likely to be removed.

The message to take from this chapter is that you should be screened for colon cancer. How you do so is open to discussion between you and your doctor, but remember that testing is important.

Resources

INTERNET

See the websites for the American Cancer Society and the National Cancer Institute already listed at the end of chapter 1 for further information about colon cancer screening in your area.

BOOKS

Adrouny, A. Richard. *Understanding Colon Cancer.* Jackson: University of Mississippi Press, 2002.

Avon, Jeffrey, M. *Gut Check: Your Prime Source for Bowel Health and Colon Cancer Prevention.* Bloomington, IN: 1st Books Library, 2001. Also available to download.

Levin, Bernard. *Colorectal Cancer.* American Cancer Society. New York: Random House, 1999.

Magee, Elaine. *Tell Me What to Eat to Help Prevent Colon Cancer.* Franklin Lakes, N.J.: New Page Books, 2001.

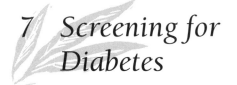

7 Screening for Diabetes

Diabetes is a very common disease in the United States today. It is estimated that 40 percent of the adult population is diabetic or prediabetic. The vast majority of those who have diabetes have what we call Type 2 or adult-onset diabetes. In this condition, which can be familial, the amount of insulin that the pancreas can produce to metabolize or burn the fuel supplied by our calories is insufficient to supply the mass of body tissue making demands upon it (as in obesity). Another aspect of Type 2 diabetes may be loss of sensitivity or ability to respond to insulin by the tissues. *Insulin* is a hormone produced by the pancreas and is necessary for your body to utilize the calories that you ingest. We most commonly hear of it affecting only carbohydrate (sugars and starches) metabolism, but its effect is much broader. If you have too little insulin or if your cells cannot recognize and use insulin, the end effect is that you pee out a lot of your carbohydrate calories and burn your muscles for body fuel. Thus, the commonly used terms "sugar diabetes" or "I've got sugar" are misleading.

Some ethnic groups are at even higher risk than the general population. These include American Indians, Polynesians, and people of native Hawaiian or Alaskan descent, to mention a few. In the United States, we are indebted to these segments of the population for participating in diabetes research, which we hope will ultimately lead to a cure for this devastating illness.

Rachel Morris Rice is a member of the Mohawk tribe of New York State. Last year she was diagnosed with diabetes. Janine, her daughter, recently came home in tears; she had just had a physical for college and the college required a blood sugar test. The nurse had told Janine that her blood sugar was elevated and that she may be prediabetic. The doctor told her to come back for fasting blood work.

"Oh, Mama, what's going to happen to me? Do I have to take medicine or give myself insulin shots? Will I get ulcers on my feet? Or go blind?"

Janine was terrified. She had grown up hearing all the bad things that diabetes can do to a person because many relatives had the disease.

The next week, Janine went back to the doctor's office early one morning having fasted from the night before, and had blood drawn for two tests: a fasting blood sugar and a Hemoglobin A_1c. To her relief, both were within the normal range. Dr. Gutierrez, her doctor, said maybe it was a good thing that her sugar had been up the other day. It signaled that she probably doesn't process her calories in the most efficient way and that unless she changes some lifestyle habits, she might become diabetic. He told her that she is prediabetic and referred her to the hospital dietitian to discuss a healthier diet. He also strongly encouraged

---

Positive Prevention of Diabetes

- In 2004, American women gynecologists from the American College of Obstetricians and Gynecologists overwhelmingly endorsed obesity as the number-one health problem facing American women.
- Obesity is directly linked to the development of diabetes.
- The United Kingdom is taking action to limit the advertising of junk food to children—a direct response to the growing problem of obesity in children.
- The United States has a true epidemic of obesity; Type 2 diabetes in children was virtually unknown just thirty years ago.
- Sensible diet and regular exercise are the best ways to deal with this important health care problem.

her to take up an active sport or pastime such as walking. Janine always enjoyed swimming, so she decided right then and there that she would join the college swim team.

Ideally, doctors would use a simple, cost-effective screen to check blood sugar levels on all patients at least once a year as is routinely done in the Indian Health Service, where awareness of diabetes is extremely high. Any single random (not fasting) blood sugar result of over 200 mg/dl (milligrams per deciliter) or at least two fasting blood sugar levels over 140 mg/dl are diagnostic of diabetes. These simple blood tests meet all the criteria for screening tests discussed in chapter 1.

Rachel, Janine's mom, learned that she has diabetes in a recent visit to her doctor. Dr. Szot had just finished doing Rachel's annual Pap exam and Rachel had finished dressing. "Rachel, I've known you now for about five years, and each year your weight has gone up a little. Last year, your blood pressure hit the bor-derline high levels and your blood fats were high. Recently, I read about a condition called Syndrome X or Metabolic Syndrome, and I realize that it fits you. You are overweight, have high blood pressure, and your blood fats—especially the triglycerides—are high. Triglycerides reflect how well your body processes total calories. In addition, I know from your history that your chil-dren weighed more than ten pounds at birth. Having all of these risk factors, you probably have impaired glucose (sugar) metab-olism and the decreased insulin sensitivity that goes with it. Let's check a two-hour glucose tolerance test to see if you handle carbohydrates in a normal way."

One week later, Rachel went to the hospital lab. She hadn't had breakfast and she was given a terribly sweet cola-tasting drink. It was all she could do to swallow it; it was just too sweet. Her blood was taken at intervals over the next two hours, and then she went home to eat a decent breakfast and have a cup of coffee. The next day, she went back to Dr. Szot and learned that her glucose toler-ance test was abnormal. Her blood sugar shot up to 200 mg/dl af-ter the syrupy drink and hovered nearly as high two hours later.

"The good news, Rachel, is that I think you can handle this with diet and exercise alone. I'm glad we checked for it before you actually had symptoms. I'm going to send you to the diabetic educator and the dietitian; they can help you make a realistic plan to change your eating habits and increase exercise. I want to see you back in one month, and I'd like to see that you have lost about five pounds."

Through awareness and simple screening, both Janine and Rachel's problems were diagnosed early, before they had symptoms and while they could favorably affect their health by lifestyle modification. This is the ideal result of screening tests and is the reason we do them.

The HgbA$_1$c (hemoglobin A$_1$c) is another blood test that is done to monitor diabetes. It isn't done as a screening test, although some doctors use it when a person has a single high blood sugar. This test tells more about sustained control of blood sugars over time, as much as three months, and is obviously useful in tracking diabetes or in evaluating whether a single elevated blood sugar result is an isolated phenomenon or if the person truly has a problem.

You may still find people who believe that we screen for diabetes by testing for sugar (glucose) in the urine. While this was true about fifty years ago, it is no longer the case. Blood sugar has to be about 180 mg/dl or higher for the average person to have glucose in their urine. We don't want to have to wait for it to be that high. In addition, some people have a lower threshold at which their kidneys spill sugar; we don't want to label all of them as diabetic. Since we now have accurate and quick methods to test blood glucose (sugar) as opposed to urine, we use blood sugar as the standard test.

Who is considered at high risk? If you meet two or more of the following risk criteria, please see your doctor for screening:

- You are obese. For adult women, this means you have a body mass index (BMI) of greater than 30 or are more than

Body Mass Index (BMI) for Women

The formula to determine BMI is: height in meters squared divided by weight in kilograms.

A BMI under 19 = underweight
19–26 = normal weight
26–30 = overweight
Over 30 = obese

Accurate scales that electronically measure BMI by bio-impedance are now widely available.

20 percent over the ideal weight for your height. For children, this means that their weight/height ratios (on the standard growth charts) are above the 85th percentile or that their BMI exceeds the 85th percentile for their age and sex. Obese little girls are at much greater risk of diabetes than are little boys.

- You have a family history of Type 2 diabetes in a first- or second-degree relative. A first-degree relative would be your father, mother, sister, or brother. A second-degree relative is an aunt, uncle, grandparent, or first cousin.
- You have Syndrome X, also known as Metabolic Syndrome.
- You have polycystic ovary syndrome.
- You have high blood pressure.
- You have high blood fats.
- You have acanthosis nigrans, a condition in which you have patches of velvety darkening of your skin.
- You or your family or ancestors are American Indian, Alaskan Native, Asian Pacific Islander, African American, or Hispanic.

Remember that identifying a problem does not give you the problem; it gives you a chance to take therapeutic measures to prolong your life and improve the quality of that life. Do not let fear be a barrier to screening.

Resources

INTERNET

The American Diabetes Association website, *www.diabetes.org,* gives information about the association, further details about different types of diabetes, diagnosis, long-term management, and resources in your community. It also offers a guide to publications, free newsletters, and tips for healthy living.

BOOKS

Bernstein, Richard, M.D. *Dr. Bernstein's Diabetes Solution.* Boston: Little, Brown, 1997.

Drum, David, and others. *The Type 2 Diabetes Sourcebook.* New York: McGraw-Hill, 2000.

Rubin, Alan, M.D. *Diabetes for Dummies.* Indianapolis, IN: Hungry Minds, Inc., 1999.

8 *Screening for Heart Disease*

Women are very aware of the risks of breast cancer, but often don't realize that heart disease is our number-one killer. We don't do walkathons to aid in the search for a cure for heart disease in women, nor do we wear little ribbons symbolizing our awareness of this most devastating illness. For some reason, we tend to think of heart disease as being a man's problem; it is, but it is equally our problem. We need to be proactive in knowing the risk factors for cardiac disease and how to evaluate our own individual risk. Statistics for the year 2000 tell us that there were 180 cardiac deaths per 100,000 women; breast cancer claimed 30 of every 100,000 women.

Jean Morris and her sister Beverly went to school with Karen Van Loon. Karen was always the life of the party, vivacious and gregarious. Last week, they heard that Karen had died of a fatal heart attack. She was fifty-four.

When you go to the doctor for your annual health checkup, you should plan to have a well-woman exam, which is a complete physical examination, not just a breast and pelvic exam. The visit should start with your completing either a specific risk assessment or a patient questionnaire, such as you find in the appendix. Risk factors can be picked up in both parts of the exam.

What are the flags that indicate increased risk? They are:

- Obesity, specifically central obesity, or being an apple instead of a pear in shape. Recent studies have indicated that a waist measurement in excess of 35 inches, or 88 cm, is a risk factor.

- Having a first-degree male relative who had a heart attack younger than age fifty-five or a first-degree female relative younger than sixty-five.
- High blood pressure. This is defined as having a systolic (top number) blood pressure higher than 140 mmHg or a diastolic (bottom number) higher than 90 mmHg. Both numbers are important. If the top number is consistently between 130 and 140 and/or the bottom number is between 80 and 90, you are considered prehypertensive.
- Smoking.
- Elevated blood fats (lipids).
- Diabetes.
- Sedentary lifestyle.

Obviously, some of these risks are screened by answering the questionnaire. Others, such as your weight and waist size, are measured with very simple, nontechnical tools, available in most homes. Blood pressure screening is done routinely in doctors' offices; in some, it may be done at each visit, in others it is done periodically. Diabetic women have a much greater risk of cardiovascular disease.

Blood fats are measured by a simple blood test. To be most accurate, the blood needs to be drawn after you have fasted for ten to twelve hours (overnight is usually adequate, unless you are a night eater).

To check blood fat levels, your doctor may order a "lipid test" or a "cardiac risk assessment panel." Your doctor is looking at your cholesterol, more properly called total cholesterol, your triglycerides, HDL, and LDL. HDL stands for high-density lipoprotein, and LDL stands for low-density lipoprotein. The total cholesterol includes LDL and HDL. We hope that your total cholesterol is not higher than 200 mg/dL. The LDL is "bad" cholesterol—the part that forms plaque on your artery walls.

Ideally, we want to see a low LDL, preferably below 160 mg/dL. How much lower depends on your other risk factors. HDL, the "good" cholesterol, is the one that tends to keep fats dispersed in the circulating blood and not clogging arterial walls. We want this to measure more than 40 mg/dL. Triglycerides are most directly affected by unwise eating and levels over 200 mg/dl can predict diabetes. Although not given proper attention until recent years, they are recognized now as part of the Metabolic Syndrome or Syndrome X that is so tightly associated with the epidemic of obesity and diabetes in the United States and other developed countries.

After these simple risk evaluations, we can group people as low risk, medium risk, or high risk. A low-risk person

- does not smoke
- has a relatively healthy family history
- has a normal blood pressure
- has normal blood fats
- does not have diabetes, and
- does not have central obesity.

A medium-risk person

- does not have diabetes, but
- may have one or two other risk factors.

A high-risk person

- is over sixty-five and has three or more of the risk factors listed above
- is diabetic, or
- already has coronary artery disease.

If a woman is low risk, the risk assessments already done are enough. If she is at medium risk, she should institute lifestyle and medical interventions to reduce her risk level. We'll discuss these later in this chapter.

If you are at high risk, more evaluation is in order, including an electrocardiogram, if not already completed. It is important to realize that an electrocardiogram (ECG, EKG) is often quite normal in a woman who is high risk but has not had a heart attack or other heart damage.

An EKG is usually done in your doctor's office. It is quick, involves no discomfort, and is relatively inexpensive. You rest on the exam table with your chest exposed. The nurse or technician applies little electrodes to your chest wall (with older versions, electrodes are also applied to the ankles and wrists). These are like small sticky Band-aids. She then attaches wires to the electrodes; these wires lead to the EKG machine, which in turn reads the electrical impulses made by your heart. A stylus records the electrical waves on a piece of paper, and the printout is called an electrocardiogram. Many machines are computer programmed to interpret the electrical impulses and "read" your EKG instantly. A doctor always reviews the EKG, for although it often is not especially helpful in evaluating risk, it is necessary in order to know whether it is safe for you to undergo some type of exercise testing.

You may have heard of certain blood tests that can help assess a person's risk of heart disease. One of these measures levels of a substance called C-reactive protein, and some experts have proposed it as being more sensitive for women's risk of heart disease than for men's. C-reactive protein is a substance produced in many parts of the body as part of the process of inflammation, and it is not specific to the heart. Blood levels of C-reactive protein are usually looked at in conjunction with measurements of another chemical substance, called homocysteine. Many doctors use these tests for individuals at medium risk of heart disease, to help in their overall assessment of such people. However, C-reactive protein and homocysteine levels are not widely used as screening tests for the general population.

A raised homocysteine level is something which can run in families. If it is known to occur in your family, or if you have a family history of heart disease, there is a simple test to detect whether or not you also have the tendency to have an elevated level. In practice the test is often omitted because getting supplemental folic acid in the diet, which is simple to add and has numerous benefits (described in chapter 17), helps lower high homocysteine levels. Two new markers are also coming into use as predictors of heart disease risk—ML (methyl peroxidase) and GP1 (glutathione peroxidase). We'll probably be hearing more of blood tests for these in the near future.

For people at medium or higher risk, a stress test is usually advised. A stress test does just what it implies: stresses the heart and allows an evaluation of whether there is hidden or potential heart disease and, if there is, how bad it is.

When you have a stress test, you are hooked up to an EKG machine by electrodes, and an initial EKG is done to establish a baseline. Usually, an oxygen sensor is attached to your index finger—kind of like having a clothespin on your finger—to check for the saturation of oxygen in your capillary blood as you exercise. You then start walking on a treadmill or, occasionally, riding a stationary bike. Meanwhile, the EKG is monitoring your heart, the oxygen sensor is measuring your oxygen saturation, and your blood pressure is being continuously recorded. At periodic intervals, the rate of exercise is increased. The exercise continues until you reach a predetermined heart rate, become fatigued, or develop symptoms such as chest pain, shortness of breath, or lightheadedness. The EKG strip is evaluated for changes that indicate lack of oxygen to the heart muscle and, therefore, increased risk of heart attack. If you experience changes such as chest pain, this is considered a suspicious stress test, even if there are no diagnostic changes on the EKG, and further evaluation is called for.

An exercise stress test is useful in evaluating whether or not you are at high risk for a heart attack and determines a safe level of exercise for you. It is also useful in assessing recovery of the heart muscle after a heart attack or any bypass or angiography procedure.

Combining an exercise stress test with a nuclear perfusion study can enhance its accuracy. In this test, a radioactive contrast substance, such as thallium or Cardiolite (also known as sestamibi) is infused into your veins prior to the test and X-rays are taken of the heart during exercise. This allows a better visualization of areas of the heart that are not adequately supplied with blood.

If a person cannot exercise because of some other illness or condition, a drug such as dobutamine or persantine can be used to stimulate the heart and mimic the effects of exercise.

Another variation is the exercise echocardiogram, a stress test with the added component of an echocardiogram, or picture of heart muscle activity, using sound waves to image the heart. This has the advantage of being able to evaluate the effectiveness of the heart muscle and valves, as well as the coronary arteries.

Conventional exercise stress tests result in more false positives in women than in men, and both exercise echocardiography and perfusion stress testing are thought to be more accurate tests for women. In some centers, your family doctor can order these tests; in others, you first need to be seen by a cardiologist.

Jean and Beverly went together to have their blood fats checked. Their father, Pop, died suddenly from a heart attack when he was just sixty. Neither had had a blood lipids check for some years, but hearing about Karen was a wake-up call. Jean knew that her high blood pressure was a risk, but it had been well controlled by medication for a long time. Beverly was a bit chunky, but mostly in the "saddlebags," not the waist. Neither had ever smoked and they had been walking together twice a week for several years.

One week later, both Jean and Beverly received the welcome news that they had very low cardiovascular risk based on their levels of blood fats. What a relief!

So, how do you minimize your cardiovascular risk? A good diet and regular exercise is a "heart smart" start. Several studies have confirmed the value of a diet high in vegetables and fruits— a pleasant way to approach this. Folic acid (folate), found particularly in dark green, leafy vegetables, is known to be essential for heart health. If needed, folic acid in the form of low-cost tablets can be used as a dietary supplement (up to a maximum of 5 mg daily). Some enjoyable physical activity done thirty minutes per day, at least five days per week is also advised. We say enjoyable because you are more likely to make exercise a nonnegotiable part of your life if you do something that you enjoy. Jean and Beverly are fortunate in having each other's companionship, and they have added tennis in good weather and squash in bad weather to their walking regimen. Previously devoted couch potatoes, they find that they love these activities.

Preventive measures you can take to ensure a healthy heart:

- Eat five to ten servings of fruits and vegetables daily.
- Exercise at least thirty minutes, at least five days a week.
- Control high blood pressure.
- Control high blood fats.
- Control diabetes.
- Don't smoke.
- Maintain a healthy weight.
- Talk with your doctor regularly about your health risks and a program to minimize them.

Resources

INTERNET

The American Heart Association provides an excellent general website, *www.americanheart.org,* for information about heart disease, minimizing risks, dealing with the immediate concerns and consequences of heart attack and stroke, tips for healthy living, and details about obtaining helpful publications. In addition, *www.womenamericanheart.org* gives specific advice for women through feature stories, self-help articles, details on resources available in your community, and information about their awareness program for women—Go Red for Heart.

BOOKS

American Heart Association. *To Your Heart: A Guide to Heart-Smart Living.* New York: Random House, 2001.

McGowan, Mary. *Heart Fitness for Life.* New York: Oxford University Press, 1999.

Sauvage, Lester. *You Can Beat Heart Disease.* 3rd ed. Seattle: Better Life Press, 2002.

9 Screening and Testing for Communicable Diseases

What is meant by the term communicable diseases? These are infectious diseases caused by bacteria, viruses, parasites, or other organisms that can be spread among the people of a community by different forms of person-to-person contact. Good examples are influenza, tuberculosis (TB), and sexually transmitted diseases. Influenza is a viral infection that is easily and rapidly transmitted from one person to another during an outbreak, as the virus travels in droplets that are coughed and sneezed into the air we all breathe. Tuberculosis is caused by bacteria that spread much more slowly than the influenza bug among people who live or work together. Sexually transmitted infections require sexual or other very intimate contact between people to spread.

It's clear from these few examples that communicable diseases can greatly impact people's health. For this reason we attach particular surveillance and control measures to such illnesses. These include, but are not limited to, screenings for preemployment and before school admittance, as well as documentation of immunity to certain diseases prior to beginning school or employment. Government employment, hundreds of occupations, and educational establishments all have different requirements for health screening for new recruits, employees, or students, and are affected by varying federal, state, and municipal regulations, which are beyond the scope of our book. Clearly, we often need to screen for or diagnose these illnesses for our own individual well being. While not encyclopedic in scope, this chapter covers the more commonly encountered infectious, or communicable, diseases and the screening procedures used to detect them.

Janine wants to be a nurse. She just took a part-time job at the hospital near her college in order to add work-related experience to her nursing program application. She was required to give evidence of immunization against rubella (German measles), hepatitis B, and polio. She had no problem doing this, as she had just updated her immunizations for college admission. The hospital also requires a screening test for tuberculosis for all of its employees. This was her first exposure to employment screening for infectious diseases.

Janine had to go to the occupational health nurse on the Monday prior to beginning work. The nurse injected a small volume of purified protein derivative (PPD) just under the skin on Janine's forearm. PPD comes from a culture of the bacterium that causes tuberculosis, *Mycobacterium tuberculosis*. It formed a little bump under the skin of her forearm, but it didn't hurt or redden. She was told to see the nurse in forty-eight to seventy-two hours for the test to be "read," which means checking for any area of hard, raised redness. In order to be considered worrisome for TB, this area needs to measure at least 10 millimeters, or about one-third inch. The reading must be done by a qualified health care professional because they are trained to evaluate ambiguous findings and know how to follow up.

Janine's test was negative—in fact, the spot had totally disappeared by the time she awakened the next day—but if it had been positive, other tests would have been done to confirm TB. These follow-up diagnostic exams include a chest X-ray and sputum (phlegm) cultures. The X-ray may show the characteristic findings of tuberculosis, which can be read by the radiologist. The sputum cultures are obtained from samples gathered from a spontaneous productive cough, by inducing the cough by a respiratory therapy technique, or by obtaining a specimen directly through a bronchoscope. The latter is a highly skilled procedure carried out by a doctor who specializes in either lung or ear, nose, and throat disease.

However it is obtained, the sputum specimen is tested in two different ways. First, a particular stain is applied that enables a trained lab technician, looking through a microscope, to identify the tuberculosis bacterium. Second, it is grown, or cultured, on a special nutrient medium that encourages the tuberculosis bacteria to grow, while discouraging the growth of other bugs.

Tuberculosis screening is required of all health care workers and people who work in health care facilities, schools, and related facilities.

Most schools and institutions of higher education, as well as health care facilities, require proof of immunity to the rubella virus in any person born after 1956; if the person cannot produce proof of immunization, a blood test can be done to test for the presence of rubella antibodies indicating that the person does have immunity. This is important to public health because rubella is dangerous to a fetus in the first few weeks of pregnancy, causing blindness, deafness, heart defects, and delayed intellectual development. The aim of rubella screening is to protect unborn children whose mothers may be exposed to the rubella virus even before they know they are pregnant. We know that in women who have immunity from rubella, these specific defects in their babies do not occur.

Screening for HIV is certainly good common sense in a society in which most people have more than one sexual partner during their sexually active years. While there is no universal guideline for this, the consensus is that it should be offered to all people, but usually is not required. Screening in prenatal clinics means that the mother can be offered certain drugs and the possibility of delivery by cesarean section if her test is positive—all measures that decrease the chances of transmission of the virus to her baby. And of course she, too, can be offered treatment. Since 1985, all blood supplied for medical purposes has been screened for HIV.

The initial test done for HIV is an antibody test; it is very good at picking up antibodies, but may produce false positives. Because of this, whenever the initial antibody test is positive, the lab performs a more expensive and time-consuming—but more accurate—test called a Western blot. If the results are equivocal, a further test called the polymerase chain reaction may be done to test for the virus itself instead of antibodies to the virus. This is highly accurate. Having just had a flu or tetanus shot may confuse these initial antibody tests, so be sure to let it be known if you have just had either shot.

The blood supply in the United States is also screened for hepatitis B and C. Many health care facilities may require their workers to be screened for hepatitis B and subsequently immunized if they are not immune. Hepatitis C is not otherwise routinely screened in the general population because there is no vaccine to offer. However, two populations are screened for Hepatitis C: illicit drug users, so that early treatment and surveillance can be offered; and frequently, pregnant women receive screenings in prenatal checks, so that if positive, the baby as well as the mother can be followed.

Many family planning clinics and other facilities offering health care for women routinely screen for gonorrhea and chlamydia infections. This is done by simple swab taken from the cervix at the time of a Pap smear and tested for DNA markers of these two illnesses. Alternatively, a "first-catch" specimen of urine can be used for this testing. Chlamydia is one of the most common causes of infertility and can be simply treated by antibiotics when identified in a timely manner. Chlamydia is increasingly prevalent in the United States and elsewhere. Gonorrhea, a cause of pelvic inflammatory disease and possible later infertility, is also eminently treatable. If a woman tests positive for these sexually transmitted diseases, we test for their bedfellows: syphilis and HIV. You may feel insulted that your doctor wants to test for these diseases, but remember that every partner brings his or her entire history to that sex act. Current monogamy may mean nothing if there is a wee virus or bacteria lurking around from previous encounters. Screening tests are meant to help you stay healthy; we are on your side!

Many states used to require a premarital test for syphilis. This is a blood test that initially tests for antibodies to syphilis; and if positive, as with the HIV test, the blood is subjected to further diagnostic testing. Premarital testing is not done as widely anymore (well, marriage is not so common either), but prenatal screening for syphilis is done with all initial prenatal testing. Syphilis is devastating to a baby who contracts the disease in the womb, as well as to any untreated individual; fortunately it can be treated with antibiotics.

In the Southwest, a Hanta screen can be done on any patient who has a high fever, flu-like symptoms, and a low platelet count on initial complete blood count. This is a quantitative platelet count and is not truly diagnostic. Timing is critical for detection of the Hanta virus: if it is suspected and the screen lends credence to that suspicion, the person needs intensive care as soon as possible.

Most people are aware of the rapid strep test that reports with reasonable accuracy within five minutes whether or not a child has strep throat. This, like many rapid tests, is based upon an antibody reaction. Because there can be false negatives, it is backed up with a true culture, meaning that the swab is stroked across a gel growth medium on which the bacteria, if present, will grow. This is the definitive diagnostic test for strep; and usually, a double swab is done on children so that no strep infection is missed in this vulnerable group. Whenever there is an outbreak of strep in a community, we may do rapid screening tests on the siblings and playmates of infected children, even if those children do not have symptoms. We may do the same with other family members if a child has repeated strep infections . . . trying to determine if a family member is a carrier of strep or, in other words, if a well person has strep living in his or her throat.

Table 9.1 Screening Tests for Common Infectious Diseases

Disease	Test
Tuberculosis	PPD (Mantoux) skin test
Rubella (German measles)	Blood test for antibody titer
Urinary tract infection	Urinalysis for WBC, RBC, protein, nitrite
Streptococcal throat infection	Rapid test for strep
Group B strep in pregnancy	Vaginal culture
HIV	Blood test for HIV antibody
Chlamydia	Cervical swab for Chlamydia DNA testing
Gonorrhea	Cervical swab for GC DNA testing
Syphilis	Blood test (RPR)
Hepatitis B	Blood test for hepatitis B antigen/antibody
Infectious mononucleosis	Blood test for antibodies

In late pregnancy, swabs are taken from the mother's vagina to culture for Group B strep. This is done because neonatal infection with Group B strep is a leading cause of neonatal morbidity and mortality. If the mother is colonized with Group B strep, she will be treated with antibiotics in labor (because the disease is very sensitive to penicillin).

In recent influenza outbreaks, with the advantage of rapid tests (based on immunologic testing), we have known certainty when we are dealing with flu. This is important because drugs are available that can shorten the duration of the flu, but they must be given within the first forty-eight hours and are not free of side effects, so we want to be sure of correct diagnosis. It is also helpful in public health tracking of the illness. These tests give us an answer within about half an hour, whereas more involved tests can take anywhere from a couple of days to a couple of weeks. By that time, the person is most likely to be either on the road to recovery or to have developed complications. Rapid tests are performed in a local lab on swabs taken from the back of your nose and throat. The longer tests are performed at reference labs on blood samples.

Diagnostic Tests for Common Infections/Infestations

Frannie went away for a camping weekend with a friend. The day after she returned, she began to have stomach cramps, followed by diarrhea. Pepto Bismol helped some, but the diarrhea didn't really stop. After a week of on-again, off-again diarrhea, she went to see Dr. Hatch, who noted that Frannie's weight was down by one and a half pounds since her well-woman visit—maybe a co-incidence, or maybe it was due to the diarrhea. Since it had already had been a week and Frannie had tried appropriate measures to stop the diarrhea, Dr. Hatch ordered stool studies for culture, ova, parasites, and antibodies to *Clostridium difficile*. She told Frannie that the latter problem was unlikely since that's the diarrhea generally caused by taking certain antibiotics, but she wanted to cover all bases.

The stool samples were examined under a microscope for any parasites or their eggs (ova). There was an almost immediate "hit." Frannie had the relatively common parasite Giardia, often found in ponds and streams, especially those frequented by beavers, but sometimes even found in municipal water supplies. In Frannie's case, this was a souvenir of her camping trip and an ill-advised slurp of water from a small stream.

If Frannie had traveled abroad, there might have been a possibility of finding other parasites in her stool. Round worms and pinworms are fairly common in developing countries; pin- or threadworms are pretty common among small children in this country, too. Occasionally these may be seen in the stool, but are more commonly diagnosed by examining the stool specimen in the laboratory. Scientifically speaking, these parasitic diseases are infestations, not infections.

Urine cultures are diagnostic for urinary tract infections. If you go to see your doctor complaining of the needing to pee too often, but having too little to pass and its hurting and burning when you do pee, your doctor first orders a urinalysis, looking for protein, blood, white blood cells, and nitrite. All are indicators of infection. He also sends the urine for a culture and sensitivity check if the urinalysis is suspicious of infection or if your symptoms are very convincing. A urine culture is done the same way as other cultures: the urine is scantily spread on a growth medium and allowed to grow in a warm environment for thirty-six to forty-eight hours. Little pieces of blotting paper impregnated with various antibiotics are placed on the growth medium. If the bacterium is sensitive to (can be killed by) the antibiotic, there is a halo of no growth around the piece of blotting paper. This enables us to know not only if you have a urinary infection, but also whether the antibiotic chosen (and there are several that we use as initial therapy) can actually cure your infection. If the antibiotic is not known to be effective against the particular "bug" that has grown out, we can change it.

Cultures done for any reason—wounds, abscesses, blood—follow the same principles and give us critical guidance to effective antibiotic therapy. We usually start treatment with an antibiotic that has a good probability of success, but culture and sensitivity testing gives us a definitive answer.

Janine's college friend Rosie became ill. She had extreme nausea, vomiting, diarrhea, and fatigue, accompanied by a low-grade fever. At first she and Janine, who was running errands and generally taking care of Rosie, thought that she had a "stomach bug" or food poisoning, but they were frightened when it went into the third day and Rosie felt no better. Janine took Rosie to the college infirmary. The doctor examined her and pointed out to Rosie that the whites of her eyes were yellow: "You have hepatitis; now we just need to find out what type."

Blood samples were drawn; some were used to look at the functioning of Rosie's liver and to follow her improvement over the next few days, and others were antigen and antibody tests for the different types of hepatitis. The most common types are hepatitis A, B, and C. Hepatitis A is generally contracted through food or water, and was the most likely culprit in Rosie's case. Hepatitis B is usually contracted through blood or unprotected sex; Rosie had neither of these risk factors and had been immunized against hepatitis B. Nor was it likely that she had developed hepatitis C, which is also usually blood borne. Over the next few days, the levels of enzymes made by her liver cells decreased, showing that she was improving; and to her great relief, her hepatitis antibody and antigen tests came back showing that she had hepatitis A.

It was soon Janine's turn to visit the infirmary. She had noticed very painful sores on her "private parts" and was terrified that she might have "caught something." Of course, the first question was whether there was a good possibility that she had been exposed to a sexually transmitted disease. Janine hated to admit it, but she'd had a drink too many at a party and had unprotected sex with a guy she hardly knew.

Terri, the nurse practitioner, examined the sores on Janine's labia and found that she also had some in her vagina. "The good news, Janine, is that these don't look syphilitic; the bad news is that I think you've contracted herpes." Terri then explained that she was going to swab the sores and send the swabs for a viral culture, but also that she was going to test Janine for all the common sexually transmitted diseases, because they tended to be constant companions. She said that with Janine's permission she was going to take swabs from Janine's cervix for chlamydia and gonorrhea, and do blood tests for herpes type 1 and type 2 antibodies, syphilis, and HIV.

Aunt Rachel just returned from Pennsylvania where she was visiting her other brother Arthur. Arthur was in a tizzy about Lyme disease, Rachel told Jean. He had been walking his dog in

Table 9.2 Symptoms and Tests for Sexually Transmitted Diseases

Disease	Symptoms	Test
Gonorrhea	Purulent discharge, burning	Cervical swab for DNA probe
Herpes simplex type 2	Flu-like symptoms, painful, shallow sores	Culture from sores, blood antibody levels
Human papilloma virus	Genital warts; may be no symptoms	DNA testing from liquid-based Pap smear or cervical swab
Syphilis	May be no symptoms; hard painless ulcer, rash, multiorgan symptoms in later stages	RPR blood test, confirmed if positive by direct antibody/antigen tests
Chlamydia	May be no symptoms; pelvic inflammatory disease, infertility	Swab from vagina or cervix for DNA probe
Hepatitis B	Nausea, vomiting, fatigue, jaundice	Blood tests for antigen/antibody
Trichomonas	May be no symptoms; burning discharge	Microscopy of wet swab from vagina/cervix; culture
Granuloma inguinale	Painful oozing ulcer	Biopsy or scrapings from the ulcer
Chancroid	Painful oozing ulcer, tender swollen lymph nodes	Culture from the ulcer

a grassy area, and the dog had a tick behind her ear. Art had just seen a half-hour TV special about the prevalence of Lyme disease in Pennsylvania, and he was worried. Rachel related how she convinced him to take the tick to the doctor's office, where it was sent to a reference lab for identification. The doctor pointed out that Art had no symptoms and that the tick identification would only take a few days. Art still wanted to have the blood test for antibodies to *Borrelia burgdorferi*, the bacterium that causes

Table 9.3 Diagnostic Tests for Common Infectious Diseases/Infestations

Disease	Test
Urinary tract infection	Urine culture and sensitivity
Influenza	Blood for influenza A and B titers
Hepatitis	Blood for hepatitis A, B, and C antigens and antibodies
Herpes simplex type 1 (cold sores)	Swabs for viral culture; blood test for antibodies
Measles	Blood for measles antibody titer
Mumps	Blood for mumps antibody titer
Septicemia (blood poisoning)	Blood culture
Bacterial diarrhea	Stool culture
Parasitic diarrhea	Microscopic exam for parasites or eggs
Strep throat	Culture from a throat swab
Lyme disease	Blood or spinal fluid for antibodies to *B. burgdorferi*
Tuberculosis	CXR, sputum for stain and culture
Meningitis	Blood and spinal fluid culture; bacterial antigens in spinal fluid
Pinworms	Microscope exam of tape placed against anus
Round worms (Ascariasis)	Microscope exam of stool
Giardia	Microscope exam of stool
Amebiasis (rare in the U.S.)	Microscope exam of stool
Tapeworm	Microscope exam of stool
Malaria	Microscope exam of blood smear

Lyme disease. The doctor tried to tell him that diagnosis of Lyme disease is not easy, even with these blood tests, and unless the tick is identified as a deer tick, he should not worry. Art worried anyway. The tick came back as a garden-variety wood tick, and Art's antibody test was, of course, negative.

Hannah had a urinary infection early in her pregnancy and after the antibiotic was finished, she began to itch. She itched so badly that she was unable to keep her hands away from her crotch and soon rubbed it raw. Dr. Seip took a look and told Hannah that it looked characteristic of yeast or candida infection, then took a swab from Hannah's vagina, and put it in a small amount of saline. She put a drop of this on a glass slide and looked at it under the microscope, after which she informed Hannah that the initial impression was correct: Hannah had a yeast infection.

Many communicable diseases can be prevented or limited in their spread by simple public health and hygiene measures. Washing hands, careful food preparation, staying home when ill, attention to pets, and other common sense measures all play a part in reducing the spread of infectious disease; and practicing safe sex goes a long way toward preventing the transmission of STDs. See chapter 17 for other methods of disease prevention, including keeping immunizations up-to-date.

Resources

INTERNET

The Centers for Disease Control's website, *www.cdc.gov*, provides extensive information about a wide range of infectious diseases and health tips for travelers, including recommended vaccines and ways to stay healthy.

10 *Screening for Bone Loss*

Beverly and Jean belong to a women's book club. The club recently read and discussed a current best-seller on osteoporosis. Since their mother died at a relatively young age of colon cancer, and they have no maternal aunts, Bev and Jean don't know if they have inherited a family risk. All fired up to check their bone strength, they enlisted Rachel and all three went to a local pharmacy that was advertising a "quick, non-invasive screen for bone loss, at a nominal fee."

What is osteoporosis? Simply put, it is the loss of bone mass and the weakening of bone structure, leading to fragile bones and an increased risk of fractures, or broken bones. Bones naturally deteriorate with age, but with detection and treatment of osteoporosis, bones can be protected and prevented from breaking.

Osteoporosis is primarily, although not exclusively, a problem of women—specifically, women over age fifty. This is because after menopause, women's levels of the hormone estrogen, which maintains healthy bones while we are younger, drop dramatically. In men, testosterone has the same function as estrogen on bones, and as men age testosterone levels do fall, but much more slowly and less dramatically than estrogen levels in women. White and Asian women are at highest risk, although African American and Hispanic women are not spared.

Osteoporosis is responsible for more than one and a half million fractures each year, and half of all women over the age of fifty can expect to have an osteoporosis-related fracture, if they are not diagnosed and treated for this problem. Unfortunately, like many of the problems for which we screen, osteoporosis is usually silent until a woman loses significant bone mass and either suffers a fracture, loses noticeable height, or develops a "widow's hump" from the collapse of vertebrae. She may also suffer severe back pain from the collapse of vertebrae.

A woman can lose as much as 20 percent of her bone mass in the first five to ten years after menopause.

Being female is not the only risk factor; other important ones are:

- Personal history of a fracture
- Family history of fractures or osteoporosis
- Being thin or small-boned
- Low bone mass
- Menopause, either natural or surgically induced
- Being older than fifty
- Long periods of no menses (except if on birth control pills)
- Eating disorders
- Certain medications, such as steroids
- Low calcium intake
- Sedentary lifestyle
- Tobacco smoking
- Alcoholism
- and, as previously mentioned, being an Asian or Caucasian woman.

Fractures due to osteoporosis are a major public health problem, as they result in a direct cost to the American public of approximately $47 million every day (2001 figures) for hospitalization and subsequent nursing home care. For many elderly women, a fractured hip is the proximal cause of death, with the final event being an infection like pneumonia, an embolism, or some other related complication.

The test that so excited Jean and Beverly was approved only recently as a screen for presumptive bone loss. It is a heel ultrasonogram (also referred to as a calcaneal bone density screen) that is non-invasive, cheap, and quickly administered. Rather than measuring bone density directly, it measures the flexibility of the Achilles tendon as it inserts into the heel bone. The degree of flexibility correlates well enough with bone density that the FDA approved the test as a screening, but not as a diagnostic measure. If a heel ultrasonometry indicates a probable lower bone mass, a follow-up DXA bone mineral density test is advised.

Heel ultrasonography is cheap and easy to do, and is sometimes offered in drugstores, health food stores, and at health fairs. Still, its availability remains limited; and in practice, the DXA bone mineral density test remains the most commonly used test both to screen and diagnose bone loss in the United States. (DXA is an abbreviation for central dual-energy X-ray absorptiometry.)

The DXA is done in conjunction with the medical imaging departments of hospitals or freestanding X-ray offices. It utilizes a very specialized X-ray of specified areas of the body, usually the hip and lower spine. A computer analyzes your readings and compares them to both a young norm and an age-matched norm. These comparisons give you what are called your T and Z scores, respectively. How much your score differs from these "normal" scores, and what its implications are for you, should be discussed with your own doctor. A variety of treatments and methods of preventing further bone loss are now available.

When having a DXA, you keep your clothes on. (Instructions you receive beforehand tell you not to wear anything with metal, such as clothing with eyelets for drawstrings or metal zippers, etc.) During the procedure, you lie on your back on an ordinary exam-type table with your legs up over a large foam block, so that you are in a tipped-over sitting posture. The X-ray is then taken through one hip and the lower spine. The whole exam usually takes less than twenty minutes.

A DXA exam can cost anywhere from $150 to $250, depending on where you live. Insurance coverage for this exam is generally quite good, although if you are menopausal at an unusually young age, your doctor may have to write letters of medical necessity for you. Medicare covers bone density testing.

Now we must mention the use of bone biomarkers. These are substances excreted in the urine that can be associated with accelerated bone loss. They are not useful as a screening measure for bone loss because they do not report anything about the status of your bones. Experts use these tests to help monitor response to treatment for osteoporosis, but not as any type of screening test. Beware that nonmedical practitioners sometimes use these tests and erroneously call them a screen. We think that this is a lack of understanding and not outright fraud, but urine testing is available to a lot of practitioners who cannot order more specific screens.

We stand by our belief that there is little point in screening for a problem if you cannot affect the outcome of that problem. Osteoporosis is now an eminently treatable condition, with several types of effective medications available. Certainly it is tragic for any woman to die from the complications of a broken hip, just for the want of a screening test and subsequent treatment.

Many experts in women's health advocate a screening DXA or heel ultrasound at the onset of menopause—or even earlier if you have multiple risk factors—and regularly thereafter. Talk with your doctor about the right time for you to begin testing.

Resources

INTERNET

The National Osteoporosis Foundation's website, *www.nof.org*, provides information about osteoporosis, answers to commonly asked questions, and details of local resources you can access.

The National Resource Center of the National Institutes of Health, Osteoporosis, and Related Bone Disorders' website, *www.osteo.org*, also provides a range of fact sheets, local addresses, information about new developments, and other useful details about preventing and managing osteoporosis.

BOOKS

Cummings, Steven and others. *Osteoporosis: An Evidence-based Guide to Prevention and Management.* Philadelphia: American College of Physicians, 2002.

Lane, Nancy. *The Osteoporosis Book: A Guide for Patients and Their Families.* London: Oxford University Press, 2001.

Nelson, Miriam, and others. *Strong Women, Strong Bones: Everything You Need to Know to Prevent, Treat, and Beat Osteoporosis.* New York: Perigee, 2001.

11 Vision Screening

Vision screening is not routinely done, except when you renew your driver's license. Sometimes, a vision screen or screen for glaucoma is done at health fairs, but it is rarely part of an annual physical (or well-woman) exam. You can do a screen at home by covering one eye and reading a chart (homemade is OK) placed about twenty feet away from you. Be sure you cover and check each eye. If there is a discrepancy between the eyes or if you find you are not seeing well, we recommend you have an exam by an eye care professional.

It is recommended that people have routine eye exams. Our focus is the comprehensive eye exam that you get from an ophthalmologist or optometrist, because it is more involved than a simple screening test.

Jean and Rachel went to see Dr. Wyman for their annual eye exam. Rachel has done this routinely since she turned forty, and Dr. Szot impressed on her the importance of continuing this now that she is diabetic and can have complications that show up in the eye. Jean started seeing Dr. Wyman the year she could no longer see to thread a needle with her naked eye.

The first thing Dr. Wyman does in the visit is review each woman's health history for the past year to see if she has had any illnesses or new medications that might reflect on her eye health.

Reading the eye chart comes next—a test most of us became acquainted with while in school. Remember trying to guess whether the letter was an E or an F?

Next you are asked to stare at a fixed point in the room (the doctor's ear makes a good target). While you do this, the doctor shines a light in your eyes, one at a time, and flips different lenses in front of the eye. Based on which allows you to most clearly read the line of letters, the doctor can approximate your need for lenses.

Before going on, Dr. Wyman covered each of Rachel's eyes in turn and observed how much the eye moved or didn't move to maintain the fixed target. This allowed him to ascertain the symmetry of Rachel's eye movements.

A refraction test is next. Dr. Wyman rolled an instrument called a phoropter in front of Jean's face and proceeded to flip down a series of lenses, each time asking Jean which of two choices gave her a clearer view. He continued until he had finely tuned a lens prescription. As it turned out, Jean really didn't need prescription glasses; she can get by with the nonprescription reading glasses that can be bought in the grocery or drugstore. She's glad because now she has a reason to go to her favorite boutique that sells very cute spectacles.

The slit lamp exam allows Dr. Wyman a highly magnified view of the eye's internal structures. It is like viewing the eye through a microscope. With this test, he can see if Rachel has any of the abnormalities caused by diabetes; or, in Jean's case, if her high blood pressure has caused narrowing of the blood vessels in the back of her eye. Used with the slit lamp exam, an ophthal-moscope is invaluable to evaluating eye diseases or the eye manifestations of systemic diseases.

For the slit lamp exam, you rest your chin on equipment that looks like a space age vehicle and then lean your forehead into another rest on the apparatus. Again you are invited to stare at a fixed point and a very bright light shines in your eye. Using this light and lenses like microscope lenses, the doctor can see the various structures and depths of the eye. He uses the ophthalmoscope to look at the structures in the back of your eye.

Glaucoma is a higher risk in African Americans, diabetics, and those with a family history of glaucoma. Effective screening for glaucoma is done best by eye specialists, such as ophthalmologists or optometrists, both of whom have specialized training and the necessary equipment. All diabetics require screening yearly, and African Americans need regular screening after age forty. Yearly exams after age sixty are adequate for screening other at-risk people.

Your eye care specialist may use a variety of tests to assess the pressure inside your eye, which is elevated in glaucoma. Tonometry or measure of the intraocular pressure is done by a variety of methods. Pneumotonometry, a common screening test for elevated pressure in the eye, uses a puff of air to flatten the cornea. Applanation tonometry uses a combination of a special probe to flatten the cornea to measure pressure and a slit lamp microscope to examine the eye. A drop of topical anesthetic is put on the eye so that you do not feel the probe. Many of you have had this test.

New tools allow the eye specialist to measure the thickness of the cornea and factor this thickness into calculations of eye pressure. This mostly benefits people who have borderline elevated eye pressure readings.

Perimetry, or visual field testing, is the single best test for diagnosing glaucoma. In this test, you stare at the center of a concave screen while lights flash in seemingly random fashion. If you see the light, you push a button and the computer records the pattern of flashing lights and your responses. When the test is finished, the computer printout illustrates any patterns of vision impairment. Your eye doctor interprets this and a diagnosis can be made based on the patterns of vision loss. Perimetry is not truly a screening test; usually it is done if one of the other tests indicates a suspicion of glaucoma.

Both Jean and Rachel were most relieved to find out that they had no eye disease—only arms that were too short and the need for lenses to overcome that!

12 Screening in Older Women

Although the age of sixty-five is beginning to seem quite young, let us accept that it connotes "older." While the other screens covered in this book are still relevant to women in their later years, some problems are either unique or accentuated in this population. The emphasis changes from promoting length of life to promoting quality of life; and screening for factors that affect quality of life include tests for vision and hearing, cognitive abilities, depression, urinary incontinence, impaired mobility, and, unfortunately, elder abuse.

We have discussed vision screening and the need for every woman to be screened annually. If a woman no longer has the ability to drive or book appointments, or is otherwise disabled, it falls to a caregiver, friend, or relative to make sure that she gets to the eye doctor. She does not necessarily need to see an ophthalmologist; optometrists are well trained to perform all the routine screens and to care for the more minor eye problems. Reputable optometrists are glad to refer you to an ophthalmologist if you have glaucoma, cataracts, or any other eye disease picked up on your screening tests. For many elderly, the ability to read, do hand work, and see TV gives great pleasure and should be safeguarded.

Hearing can be screened by a simple question whispered while doing a patient interview or exam. Or, a friend can rub strands of hair together by the woman's ear and see if she can hear it. If there seems to be a problem, referral to an audiologist is justified. Again, listening to a bird's song, music, or a child's voice may be among the few pleasures left to women who are alone or disabled by some chronic disease.

Growing older is a process of gradual losses: spouses, family, friends, and our own abilities. It is no surprise, therefore, that many older women become depressed. Many no longer feel needed or important to anyone and may feel that they are a burden on the people that they love. Our society has grown cold to the values of extended family and the important role elders used to play within the extended family. Now we look for nursing home placement—or, if Momma still has all her pieces intact, we call it an extended care or assisted living facility. No individual is at fault here; society has disintegrated to the extent that most families have to put all their energies into the daily maintenance of their nuclear family. Few families have the luxury of time and proximity needed to care for older loved ones.

Among the losses that many women (our mothers) sustain is the loss of trusted providers of medical care. This may be through the retirement or death of a doctor, relocation to live in a more senior-friendly community, or a move to be nearer her grown children. Unfortunately this often happens at the same time medical needs increase, needs that frequently call for more complex, high-tech procedures. Understanding these can be hard enough for younger people—for older citizens in our community they can be truly frightening. Our mothers really need our help at this time.

There are several brief questionnaires that help to assess depression. It is good care to administer these at least once a year and to be sensitive to possible depression if you hear there are complaints of fatigue, lack of interest in things she used to enjoy, or if she does not follow medical advice.

Assessing a woman's activities of daily living, including dressing herself and preparing meals, can give a fairly accurate picture of her functional capacity. Again, there are simple questionnaires that are very helpful with this assessment. A woman may not think about being functionally limited when she eats tea and toast for every meal. She may have given up cooking so gradually that it seems normal to her now. She may equally blame the rug in the room or a misplaced object for her lack of balance. It is important to realize these changes are taking place before major mishaps or illnesses occur.

Sometimes women come in and complain about the quality of their memory; more often, they do not mention the gaps in their memory, and indeed, try to cover up the lapses. Although sometimes our questions may seem insulting, it is reasonable to ask what day of the week it is, the date, the year, the names of the last three presidents as well as the current vice president. If they can't answer these questions, it is a good idea to have a more formal cognitive assessment done. If their memory is significantly impaired, they may be at high risk for mishaps.

Remember screening your home to make sure that it was childproof? Well, at the other end of life, home safety is again a big issue. You need to check the home for any hazards that may lead to a fall, install hand grips in the bathroom, make sure frequently used items are not placed on high shelves, and check the water temperature to make sure the water heater is set no higher than 125 degrees Fahrenheit. You want to make sure that walkways are kept free of snow and ice and that attractive nuisances like skateboards and roller skates are not in the path. Kettles with automatic turnoffs are a good idea. Check the smoke and carbon monoxide detectors, first to see that they are installed, and secondly, to see that they work. It is a good idea for elderly women who spend much time alone to have some type of alarm device by which they can signal 911 or the local first-response team. This has saved many lives and is worth the small monthly cost. If your beloved mother or other loved one cannot afford it—or refuses to spend the money— this would make a very loving gift.

Many women are too embarrassed to admit that they are leaking urine. You have to ask; and if the response is yes, then talk with her doctor and introduce her to the pull-ups and pads available in any supermarket. There is a good reason that there are so many products available: it is a very common problem. Go to the doctor first, though, because she may have a very treatable problem.

Elder abuse and neglect is a growing problem, as well. The more our population ages and our resources are stretched, the greater this problem becomes. Like child abuse, it happens in all strata of society and is largely hidden. It is also reportable to authorities in the same way as child abuse. In fact, in many places, the child abuse hotline is used to report elder abuse. Elder abuse may range from the extortion of "gifts" from women who are cognitively impaired to actual physical assault. It happens in private homes and in public facilities. The only way we can stop it is by first acknowledging that it is a problem and that it is increasing. Maintaining a high index of suspicion helps to detect problems, especially when asking women about things going on in their daily lives that may elicit revealing responses.

We have discussed screening for osteoporosis in a previous chapter, but reiterate the magnitude of this problem for aging women.

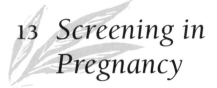

13 Screening in Pregnancy

One year ago, Frannie's cousin Jeff married Hannah, a young African American widow with two children from her previous marriage. Hannah's first husband was also African American, and while she had serious doubts about bringing her children into a mixed marriage, the warm welcome of Jeff's extended family wiped her doubts away. Jeff has never been married and wants to have at least one biological child; at thirty-six, Hannah has qualms about attempting another pregnancy. Her daughter is eight and her son ten, so there would be a big age difference if she and Jeff had a child. Finally, she resolved to let nature solve the dilemma; if she became pregnant, so be it.

When Hannah missed her period for six weeks, she went to the drugstore and bought a home pregnancy test. (Home pregnancy tests are usually the first test done in pregnancy.) In the privacy of the bathroom, she read the directions and then peed into a paper cup. Next she dipped the wand of what looked like blotting paper into the cup of urine and watched as the urine soaked the paper, moving toward the all-important test area. With mixed emotions, she saw the magical blue lines appear—a definite positive. She sprinted back to the bedroom to awaken Jeff with the news.

The test you buy may indicate a positive reading with either a red line or blue line, but all tests are based upon the same chemical principles. In each pregnant woman's urine there is a substance called beta human chorionic gonadotrophic hormone, or β-HCG for short. This is formed by the cells that become the placenta and is present very early in pregnancy. In fact, a pregnancy test is usually positive from the first day that a period is missed in a woman with a twenty-eight-day cycle.

Some precautions are necessary when you use a home pregnancy test. First, of course, is to read the directions. It is advisable to test the very first time you urinate in the morning because the urine is more concentrated after you have slept for hours without drinking. Be sure the urine is collected in a clean container and that it is not contaminated by blood for any reason. Check the date on the package; if it is out of date, the test may not be accurate. Make sure the test has not been refrigerated, and do not refrigerate your urine before doing the test. Either a cold test or cold urine can cause a false negative result. Generally these tests are very accurate and reliable, but these are two things that can trigger false negative results. If you have a negative test and still think you might be pregnant, wait a few days and then repeat the test or go to your doctor for a blood pregnancy test.

The next day, Hannah went to see her family doctor, Dr. Murphy, who did a blood pregnancy test—based on the same β-HCG—and confirmed the results of the home test. Because Hannah had had a couple of miscarriages after the birth of her daughter, Dr. Murphy also had the lab check to see how much HCG was in Hannah's urine, because a higher level is somewhat predictive of a sturdy pregnancy. The level was reassuringly high, a fact Hannah reported to Jeff with growing excitement.

Dr. Murphy referred Hannah to Dr. Seip to follow her pregnancy, and Hannah's first visit was scheduled for ten days later. It is good practice to have your first prenatal visit as early as possible and certainly within the first twelve weeks (the first trimester) of pregnancy. For Hannah this was even more important because she had the additional risk factors of being over age thirty-five and having had two previous miscarriages. Dr. Seip had been Hannah's ob-gyn for many years and was well aware of these factors.

Dr. Seip looked over Hannah's updated patient questionnaire to make sure that she was not suffering any problems other than mild morning sickness and, specifically, that she had had no spotting or bleeding since her last period. She then had Hannah undress and did a physical exam, including a pelvic exam with a Pap smear and tests for chlamydia and gonorrhea. Next, Dr. Seip put conductive gel on Hannah's belly for an ultrasound to determine the well-being of the fetus and accurate dating for the pregnancy. The ultrasound utilizes high-frequency sound waves to form an image much like an X-ray, but without the risks. Sometimes a vaginal probe rather than an abdominal one is used. The woman is usually given the probe, shaped like a tampon and covered with a condom, to insert into her own vagina. In many cases the vaginal probe, being closer to the uterus and other pelvic organs, transmits clearer ultrasound pictures than the abdominal one.

Ultrasound is used in early pregnancy for a number of reasons. First, it is the most accurate way to date a pregnancy because in the earliest stages of pregnancy babies tend to be the same size in their stage of development. After the halfway mark of the pregnancy, each baby grows in its own individual manner and there can be great variability. We all know that babies can weigh anywhere from six to ten pounds at birth and be perfectly normal. Knowing accurate dates can be important, especially if there are any risk factors that may influence the progress of the pregnancy and how it is followed. Ultrasound also tells us whether there is a single fetus present, or two, or three, or more! This is useful not only because parents want to know this as early as possible, but also because multiple pregnancies require extra medical care.

Early ultrasound is also useful for determining that a pregnancy is healthy—we use the term "viable." We can see the heart beating, and can be sure that the pregnancy is in the uterus where it belongs and not in the tubes. Hannah was thrilled and reassured to see the fuzzy gray shape of her developing baby and the visible beating of the heart on the ultrasound screen.

Having said this, it is important to realize that ultrasound at this early stage gives limited information about the long-term health of the fetus. Much can change, which is why we advise continued monitoring of pregnancies.

At the conclusion of this first visit, Dr. Seip ordered the prenatal panel of blood tests for Hannah. What is the prenatal panel? These blood tests check the mother's health and pick up any diseases that could compromise the unborn child. Tests usually included are the CBC, or complete blood count; blood glucose; blood type and Rh factor as well as antibodies that are more unusual; rubella immune status; hepatitis B and C immune status; RPR for syphilis; and a urine specimen. HIV testing is advocated, but it is not routinely done in all practices.

- CBC is done particularly to be sure that the woman is not anemic. Anemia, especially iron deficiency anemia, is a relatively common problem in young women and is important to be corrected. Red blood cells contain the iron-containing pigment hemoglobin, the vehicle by which oxygen to the developing baby, as well as to the mother's vital organs, is transported in the blood. If you don't have enough hemoglobin, you are anemic. In pregnancy although there is an increase in the number of red blood cells, there is an even greater increase in the plasma (the milky fluid in which the red and white cells float), so the available hemoglobin is diluted. This means that pregnant women normally have lower hemoglobin levels than nonpregnant women. In the first two trimesters (a trimester is about three months), we consider a woman anemic if her hemoglobin falls below 11 g/dL and in the last three months, she is anemic if it falls below 10.5. When these levels fall, we treat the woman with iron, in addition to her prenatal vitamins. These vitamins also contain the vital nutrient folic acid, which helps to prevent certain birth defects. Sometimes folic acid deficiency or vitamin B_{12} deficiency may be particularly indicated by the blood smear examined by the lab. Red cells appear larger than normal in B_{12} deficiency, whereas in iron deficiency the red cells appear smaller.

- Testing for ABO blood group is done primarily in case the woman needs a blood transfusion for any reason. Occasionally, a woman has more unusual antibodies in her blood; these are screened, so that compatible blood is available should she need it during delivery. The need for transfusion is reasonably uncommon, but we still need to be prepared for the possibility.

- Rh factor is important. Being Rh positive simply means that you have a protein called the Rhesus factor attached to your red blood cells. An Rh-negative woman does not have this protein and it has no meaning in her life unless she is exposed to Rhesus factor either by being transfused with Rh-positive blood (which all blood transfusion services make sure does not happen) or she becomes pregnant with a baby who is Rh positive. This can happen if the baby's father is Rh positive. Considering that 99 percent of Asian Americans, 95 percent of African Americans, and 85 percent of white Americans are Rh positive, this is quite likely. If during the pregnancy or labor some of the baby's red blood cells enter the mother's bloodstream, the mother may develop antibodies to Rhesus-positive red blood cells. In a subsequent pregnancy with a Rhesus-positive baby, these antibodies may cross the placenta, destroying that baby's red blood cells and causing the baby to become very anemic, and possibly causing the baby to die. In other words, the first pregnancy can act to sensitize the mother, so that later pregnancies are put at risk.

Because of this, Rh-negative women in decades past lost many babies. Today, this rarely happens because we screen mothers ahead of time and treat those at risk with an antibody (called anti-D or Rhogam) before the body begins to make its own antibodies. This treatment has revolutionized the care of Rh disease in newborns, which until the 1970s was a major cause of death. Now the antibody is given to Rhesus-negative women after they give birth to Rh-positive babies or during pregnancy, if there is any bleeding or any procedure that needs to be done which may cause a transfer of red blood cells from the baby to the mother.

There are some other much less common antibodies that can affect a baby in the same way as Rh antibodies; these, too, are routinely screened for with the prenatal panel of tests.

Hannah's hemoglobin was found to be 12 mg/dL and the rest of her CBC was normal, as well. She is very conscious of eating a good diet and includes plenty of leafy green vegetables and protein. She is Rh negative, but received Rhogam after her previous pregnancies and miscarriages, so she has not developed antibodies.

- Rubella antibody titres. Hannah was quite sure that she had immunity to rubella (German measles), but was relieved to have it tested by measuring the levels of antibodies against rubella. Having rubella in the first weeks of pregnancy can cause severe birth defects in the baby, including hearing and vision defects as well as heart problems. The advent of a vaccine against rubella has made these tragedies virtually unheard of today. Usually given in childhood, it is given when a woman enters college if she has not been vaccinated previously. Once in awhile, a woman has inadequate rubella immunity and has to protect herself against exposure during pregnancy and then be immunized after the baby is born. Hannah didn't have the vaccine because her childhood pediatrician knew that she had had the illness and her subsequent test levels proved this to be true.
- Hepatitis B is a serious blood-borne disease and is very infectious. We now offer a vaccine to all newborn infants and

are hopeful that this policy of universal immunization will eradicate the illness.

- Hepatitis C is common among drug users and sex workers. Although you may not fall into either of these categories, it is discriminatory to try to figure out who does. For this reason, it is good public health policy simply to screen all pregnant women. Many hospitals and clinics adhere to this; ask if yours does. Because hepatitis C can be transmitted to the baby, it is good to know ahead of time if the risk is present so that counseling and treatment can be offered. This test is not routinely done in all practices.

- The RPR test for syphilis is routinely done because the baby in the womb can contract this sexually transmitted disease and the effects are devastating. It makes sense to test for the disease because it can be easily treated with antibiotics. The RPR is a screening test and labs automatically confirm positive results with more specific diagnostic tests.

- Blood glucose screening is done early in many hospitals and clinics because gestational diabetes (diabetes in pregnancy) is becoming more common; if present, the sooner the mother is treated by diet and/or insulin the better for the baby. It is routinely checked again later in pregnancy.

- HIV screening has been a hot potato in many institutions. The current public policy is to encourage voluntary screening for HIV, but not to require it; check with your doctor about the practices in your particular community and state. It is very important for the baby's health to diagnose maternal HIV before delivery, if possible, because we now have drugs that prevent transmission. We also can choose to deliver the baby by cesarean section to further decrease the risk of transmission to the baby.

- Urine tests. Hannah was asked to provide a midstream urine specimen. The urine is examined for protein, glucose, and blood and a culture is done. (It is smeared on a special growth medium—kind of like Jell-O—to see whether

Table 13.1 Summary Table of Initial Prenatal Tests

Test	Condition Screened For
CBC	Anemia
Blood type and Rh factor	Possible Rh disease in the baby
Other blood antibodies	As above
Rubella antibodies	Immunity to rubella (German measles)
RPR	Syphilis
Hepatitis B surface antigen	Hepatitis B
Pap smear	Precancerous changes
GenProbe swab	Chlamydia and gonorrhea
Urinalysis	Protein, glucose, blood in urine
Urine culture	Asymptomatic urinary infection
HIV	HIV
PPD	TB

bacteria grow.) It is important to recognize any urine infection early, even if it isn't causing symptoms, because urinary infections during pregnancy can cause kidney damage or other unpleasant ill effects for the mother as well as increase the risk of premature labor.

- PPD. In geographic areas with higher tuberculosis risk, a PPD skin test is used to screen the mother for possible TB. Not universally applied in pregnancy, this test is done only in certain populations or geographic regions at greater risk, such as American Indian reservations, the inner city, and people who are occupationally exposed to patients with TB.

You have read that Hannah had a simple ultrasound in Dr. Seip's office at her first prenatal visit, but you may want to know more about the ultrasound test.

With ultrasound scanning, high frequency sound waves are transmitted into the body. Different types of tissue, for example solid versus more liquid, reflect these waves differently, allowing a two-dimensional image of deep body structures—made by these reflected sound waves—to be displayed on the viewing screen. Over the past twenty-five years, ultrasound has completely revolutionized the practice of obstetrics. Thirty years ago, all women who had bleeding in the later months of pregnancy were confined to bed for months—sometimes until their babies were born—because there was no accurate way of telling where the placenta was developing. Now we can tell this and check the baby's well-being within minutes by using a simple bedside ultrasound, as well as reassure the mother. Ultrasound has been widely used in millions of women over the past thirty years, and no adverse effects from this technology have been identified. Like most technologies, the accuracy and helpfulness of ultrasound is reliant on the expertise of the people performing and interpreting the images formed. This is gained through training and experience.

As in all screening tests, there are false positives and false negatives. The false positives suggest an abnormality that isn't really there, which leads to more tests, worry to the parents, and increased costs. False negatives fail to identify an abnormality that is there and may lead to a delay in therapeutic action. You need to be aware of these possibilities before agreeing to have an ultrasound.

The primary purpose of Hannah's initial ultrasound was to establish the accuracy of her expected delivery date. Hannah's age and previous history of miscarriage were adequate reasons for Dr. Seip to decide that Hannah should have another ultrasound at eighteen weeks of pregnancy. This is commonly, but not universally, done. This ultrasound was done in a medical imaging facility in Dr. Seip's office building and was read by a doctor specializing in ultrasound. The baby's brain, heart, kidneys, limbs, and other organs were checked with a much larger and more sophisticated ultrasound machine than the one in Dr. Seip's office. Dr. Seip explained that though these findings were very reassuring they did not imply a 100 percent guarantee of a perfectly normal baby—other possible abnormalities cannot be seen on ultrasound and conditions can develop later in a pregnancy that may interfere with a baby's health. The positioning of the placenta was also assessed in this exam. Jeff went along with Hannah to see the ultrasound done, and he was thrilled to see the baby so clearly on the screen. Both he and Hannah decided they did not want to be told the baby's sex at this stage.

The eighteen-week ultrasound also can also be useful if there is any concern about the baby's growth, which usually occurs because a woman previously has previously had a small baby. Small-for-dates babies have been found to have significant health problems in childhood. This ultrasound provides a good basis against which later growth can be measured.

Another use of ultrasound increasingly is being offered to pregnant women, in this case at the eleven- to thirteen-week stage. This test, called fetal nuchal translucency (FTN), is an exam of the tissue at the back of the developing baby's neck. It's known that babies with certain abnormalities including Down's syndrome may have a greater thickness of tissue in this area. When this measurement is made, along with two other blood tests (one a measurement of that same HCG hormone we've already mentioned, and the other a protein called PAPP-A) and the results are put into a computer, an estimate can be given of the likelihood of the baby having one of these abnormalities. It is important to understand that this is a screening test, and not a diagnosis of Down's syndrome or other abnormality. If the estimated risk is high, further tests are offered. In fact on further testing, most women who are described as high risk do not have an abnormal baby. And a proportion of those described as low risk nevertheless do give birth to a baby with Down's syndrome. The actual proportions of high- and low-risk women, in addition to the sensitivity and specificity of the tests (refer to chapter 1 for definitions) vary from one lab to another—and is specific information you need to request from your doctor. There are no risks to yourself or the baby from having these tests. FTN and associated tests are covered more fully in chapter 15.

Early in her pregnancy, Hannah began to think about whether or not to have an amniocentesis. Dr. Seip discussed the procedure with Hannah because her age posed an increased risk of her baby's having Down's syndrome. Formerly referred to as mongolism, Down's syndrome is a genetic defect in which the affected person has three of the chromosomes called number 21, instead of the normal two. (Remember that we ordinarily have one copy of each chromosome from each parent.) This is called trisomy 21, and is associated with certain physical changes and reduced intellectual development. A woman whose infant is found to have Down's syndrome in the first half of pregnancy may choose to terminate the pregnancy.

In women under age thirty-five, Down's syndrome occurs in about 1 in 600 births. After age thirty-five, the risk steadily increases with age, with about a 1 in 200 risk at age thirty-seven, 1 in 70 at forty years, and 1 in 20 at age forty-five. Because of these risks, amniocentesis is suggested to women age thirty-five and over. Hannah opted not to have an amniocentesis because she and Jeff had discussed it and decided not to terminate the pregnancy even if there was a problem, so there was no point in exposing themselves to even the small risk of miscarriage associated with amniocentesis (about 1 percent in experienced hands).

Instead, Hannah was offered and opted to do a blood test called "serum screening." This blood test is a screening offered to all women over thirty-five; many doctors now believe that either this test, or the FTN plus blood tests we've mentioned previously, should be done routinely for *all* women, since the majority of babies with Down's syndrome are actually born to younger mothers. This test measures alpha fetoprotein, estriol, inhibin, and quantitative levels of HCG. Alpha fetoprotein is a substance produced by the baby's liver and is measurable in the mother's blood. Elevated levels of this substance are suspicious of neural tube defects (relating to the spine and brain, like spina bifida) and some other abnormalities; lower levels are present in Down's syndrome. HCG is the hormone human chorionic go-nadotrophin and is made by the placenta, as is inhibin; unconju-gated estriol is one of the normal estrogens produced by women and is highest in pregnancy. Variations in the normal levels of all four of these indicate a high risk of congenital disorders. The serum screen usually is done between the fourteenth and seven-teenth weeks of pregnancy. A computer program is used to give an individual woman an estimate of her risk of having a baby with Down's syndrome. Please note that like the FTN and earlier blood tests, this is a *risk estimate*—it is a screening test and not an exact diagnosis of whether or not the baby is affected. If the serum screen test is suspicious, indicating a high risk of the baby having Down's syndrome or some less common abnormalities, a woman is offered diagnostic testing to confirm or refute these findings. Hannah's serum screen put her in the low-risk range, so she felt more secure about not having an amniocentesis done, even though she understood it was not a guarantee that her baby was unaffected.

Because Hannah had been evaluated in her first pregnancy for sickle-cell anemia and knew that she did not carry the gene, so she was not worried about that. This condition is more common in people of African descent and is usually tested for in a first pregnancy (also see chapter 16).

As you are gathering, amniocentesis is not a screening test used on all pregnant women. In fact, it is a diagnostic test, not a screening test, and is offered only to a select group of women based on their risk factors. In this test, a long slender needle guided by ultrasound imaging is passed through the abdom-inal wall and into the pool of fluid in which the baby is sus-pended. Some of this fluid is drawn off and sent to the lab to examine the chromosomes in the cells of the fluid. There is a slight risk—0.5 percent—of amniocentesis causing a miscarriage. This risk is increased if the placenta is lying just across the front of the uterus close to the place where the needle enters. The cells in the fluid sample are examined in the laboratory for the chromosomal abnormalities characteristic of Down's syndrome as well as for a variety of other possible genetic defects, such as Tay-Sachs, sickle-cell anemia, or thalassemia (another form of anemia occurring mostly in people of Mediterranean origin), if desired. Amniocentesis is done around sixteen weeks of pregnancy; and although a preliminary result is available within a few days, the complete chromosomal identification can take up to three weeks. This is important to note because if a woman chooses to terminate an affected pregnancy, it has to be done by inducing labor, a physically and emotionally distressing procedure that sometimes can last several days.

Another diagnostic test is chorionic villous sampling (CVS). This is basically a biopsy of the developing placenta that can be done between ten and twelve weeks of pregnancy. In this procedure, a sampling tube is passed through the woman's cervix under ultrasound guidance. Fetal cells are removed and can be cultured and identified within forty-eight to seventy-two hours, allowing the woman to have a reasonably simple termination of the pregnancy by dilating the cervix and suctioning of the products of conception from the uterus. This is an advantage, but there are disadvantages that also need to be considered before opting for CVS. This is an invasive test that is quite uncomfortable, however temporarily. There also is a greater risk of miscarriage than with amniocentesis, a risk of 1 to 1.5 percent even in experienced hands. Another unfortunate possibility is that enough cells may not be retrieved for accurate analysis and identification, in which case the procedure may need to be repeated or an amniocentesis done instead.

As your pregnancy advances, one of your doctor's simplest screening tools is a tape measure. The growth of your belly is measured at each visit and the results are compared against norms. Being too big too soon may signal multiple fetuses, too much fluid in the womb, or a bigger than average baby. This indicates the need to do more diagnostic procedures, such as ultrasound. Similarly, too little growth signals the need for diagnostic evaluation. If your doctor recommends it, ultrasound may be used for medical indications in the last few months of pregnancy. You should understand why this is being recommended, however. Ultrasound is not used routinely as a screening test for the progress of pregnancy at the present time.

At each visit, your blood pressure is taken; we expect pregnant women to have a low to middle-of-the range blood pressure. A high blood pressure, if persistent, may signal that the placenta is unable to adequately nourish the growing baby, and may also be a danger to the mother herself. In most places your weight is also recorded at each visit. A large weight gain may indicate problems with your health, and too little weight gain makes us suspicious that the baby is not growing properly, although there is less concern now about mother's weight than there used to be.

You may be asked to donate a urine sample at each visit. This has been customary to check for sugar or protein in the urine, but is not used as universally as it once was. There are better screening methods of screening for diabetes, and any swelling of the feet and hands or elevation of blood pressure tells us to check if you are losing protein in your urine.

After about twenty weeks, your doctor "listens" for your baby's heart at each visit. This "listening" is no longer done with a stethoscope; the doctor uses a Doppler machine, which is actually another type of ultrasound machine. The echoes that the machine picks up from the blood moving in the baby's heart are converted into audible heartbeats that you can hear. Don't be surprised or alarmed at how fast these are—usually about 120 to 140 beats per minute. This is normal. Conductive gel is put on your belly to help the small microphone in the Doppler machine pick up the magical sound of your baby's heartbeat.

Blood Tests Later in Pregnancy

With the increase in Type 2 diabetes mellitus in all developed countries, there is an increasing problem with gestational diabetes, meaning diabetes occurring only in pregnancy. Gestational diabetes is a signal that the mother may subsequently become diabetic, and it puts the baby at risk for congenital anomalies and future diabetes. Type 2 diabetes is endemic among certain American ethnic groups, including Alaskan natives, American Indians, and Polynesians, and they routinely receive early screening for diabetes. All women who are not high risk are screened between twenty-six and twenty-eight weeks, although the usefulness of this continues to be debated among doctors. Besides ethnicity, high-risk factors are: abnormal fasting blood sugar in the initial blood work; previous gestational diabetes; strong family history of diabetes; and having had a previous baby weighing more than ten pounds. The screening test employed is a random one-hour postload blood test. What does this mean? You are given 50 grams of a very sweet liquid that tastes like cola; one hour after drinking this, your blood is drawn and the glucose level is measured. If your blood sugar is higher than 140 mg/dL, you need to have a glucose tolerance test (similar to the procedure described in chapter 7). The screening load test can be done any time; the glucose tolerance test needs to be done after an overnight fast—in other words, you go to the lab or doctor's office without having any food or drink since dinner the night before. When you come for the test, you are given 100 grams of the cola drink after an initial fasting blood draw. Then your blood is drawn at one-, two-, and three-hour intervals, and the blood sugar levels are read. Acceptable levels are:

- Fasting—up to 105 mg/dL
- One hour—up to 190 mg/dL
- Two hours—up to 165 mg/dL
- Three hours—up to 145 mg/dL

Fortunately, Hannah's glucose levels were all within the normal range.

Because of her Rh-negative status, Hannah had the test again at twenty-six weeks to see if she had developed antibodies. She had not and was given 300 micrograms of Rhogam, or anti-D, at twenty-eight weeks. This is the standard approach in the United States, with slight variations in the United Kingdom and Australia. Unless the delivery is delayed more than twelve weeks after this dose, she will not be tested or receive another dose until the baby is born, at which time she'll receive another 300 micrograms anti-D if the baby is Rh positive. The American College of Obstetricians and Gynecologists (ACOG) recommends that an Rh-negative woman who has not formed antibodies should receive anti-D immune globulin:

- At about twenty-eight weeks of gestation, unless the baby's father is also Rh negative,
- Within seventy-two hours of the birth of an Rh-positive baby, and
- After a miscarriage or abortion in the first trimester.

There is consensus that anti-D should be considered if any of the following have happened:

- A threatened miscarriage,
- Second or third trimester bleeding,
- Trauma to the abdomen, or
- Attempts to turn the baby in the uterus by hands on the abdomen (usually because the baby is in the breech position).

Infections are a significant risk to newborns; if there is a possibility that you may have contracted an STD during pregnancy, be open with your doctor about this so that you can be tested again for gonorrhea, chlamydia, syphilis, and HIV.

The Centers for Disease Control (CDC) recommend a vaginal swab be taken at thirty-five to thirty-seven weeks gestation for culture to screen for Group B strep because this organism can cause much morbidity and mortality for both mother and baby. If this test shows Group B strep, penicillin or another antibiotic may be given during labor. Fortunately, Hannah's test was negative.

Pregnancy is a happy time, and the purpose of good prenatal care is to keep it happy. Screening and early detection of problems can prevent much future tragedy. We are happy to tell you that three days before her expected date, Hannah gave birth to a beautiful nine-pound boy named William Jeffrey Harris Acton—Billy to all his extended family.

Resources

INTERNET

The American College of Obstetricians and Gynecologists (ACOG) website, *www.acog.org*, provides comprehensive information about issues of interest in women's health, fact sheets and publications that cover pregnancy and pregnancy care, and information about local resources and service providers. Many of their publications of ACOG are available through your family physician or local hospital outpatient clinic.

14 *What's Left Out and Why*

Although some treatment options are available, there are three common cancers among women for which there are no simple, effective, and safe screening tests. These cancers and thyroid disease from the gland situated in the neck, which is responsible for normal metabolism and the functioning of all other body systems, are the topics of this chapter.

Lung Cancer

Rachel just lost a good friend, Betty, to lung cancer. Betty died within a few months of being diagnosed, and Rachel questioned a doctor friend very closely as to why Betty hadn't been given lung X-rays or some other form of screening. "After all, everybody knew that Betty smoked like a chimney."

We wish that a simple chest X-ray were an effective screen for lung cancer, but it is not. That is why routine chest X-ray screening has not been done for many years. If a lung cancer is picked up on a routine chest X-ray, that is a lucky coincidence; usually a lung cancer is very far advanced by the time it shows up in a nonselected population on a simple chest X-ray.

There is an ongoing research project to see if a specialized CT scan (called spiral CT scan) is able to pick up early lung cancers in a high-risk population. The National Lung Screening Trial (NLST) compares spiral-computed tomography with standard chest X-ray to see if either is an effective method to reduce deaths from lung cancer.

Interestingly, it has been noted that people who have been scanned by spiral CT scan as part of screening trials are more apt to quit smoking on a long-term basis than other smokers. One year after being scanned, 14 percent of smokers had quit smoking for good, as compared to 6 percent of the general smoking population. There was no correlation with the findings of disease, so we guess that relief was as powerful a motivator as fear.

Lung cancer is the leading cause of cancer-related death in the United States and is usually caused by exposure to tobacco smoke. Women seem to be more susceptible than men to the carcinogens in tobacco. Lung cancer is the leading cause of death for women smokers aged forty to seventy-five. Survival rates are far poorer than for breast cancer.

The NLST is recruiting fifty thousand current or former smokers for a study that lasts until 2009. People participating in the trial receive a free screening by either chest X-ray or spiral CT scan. If you wish to check your eligibility to participate, call 800 – 422 – 6237 for information in either English or Spanish.

Endometrial Cancer

Endometrial cancer (cancer of the lining of the uterus) is the most common of the gynecological cancers. If you live in the developed world and reach age seventy-five with your uterus intact, you have a 1 in 80 chance of developing endometrial cancer. In other words, this is usually a cancer of older women.

There are some definite and well-recognized risk factors:

- Obesity
- Diabetes mellitus, Type 2
- Hypertension
- Unopposed estrogen therapy, meaning no progestin is involved (This is rarely done.)

- Lack of ovulation. Women with polycystic ovary syndrome are one example. This can be a cause of endometrial cancer at a young age.
- Use of tamoxifen. This is a useful drug for breast cancer, and doctors are aware that it carries two to three times the normal risk of endometrial cancer, so women taking tamoxifen are tested on a routine basis.
- Genetic causes, including an association with certain non-polyp types of colon cancer.

There are currently no accepted screening tests for the general population of women. However, high-risk patients may be screened by ultrasound scans that measure the thickness of the endometrium (lining of the uterus) or by endometrial biopsies (taking small samples of the lining for examination under a microscope). Although they have been proposed as screens for the general population, each has significant limitations.

Ultrasound scanning of the endometrium measures the thickness of the endometrial lining, which varies with the cycle of a menstruating woman. But after menopause, in a woman not taking hormone replacement therapy, the endometrial lining usually stabilizes at 5 mm or less in thickness. Large-scale screenings of whole populations of women have been disappointing as far as the value of this test as a screen because of the large number of false positives produced. Many women (up to 50 percent) had to undergo further evaluations based on a suspicious ultrasound result, but the yield of women with cancer was low (average 4 percent).

Endometrial biopsy is done by inserting a very thin plastic tube through the opening in the cervix into the uterus to suck out a sample of the tissue lining the uterus. This procedure needs to be done by a doctor with special training and requires a speculum examination of the cervix first (as described in chapter 4). This examination is never comfortable, requires clinical expertise, may be very difficult in postmenopausal women, is costly, and may have adverse side effects. But, most importantly, it is not reliable as it obtains only a small sample of the endometrium and may miss a cancer. This does not meet the criteria for a screening test, although in clinically indicated situations it can be useful (for instance, for women taking tamoxifen).

Because of these limitations, screening by these methods should be confined to those women identified as high risk.

Ovarian Cancer

Ovarian cancer accounts for about 4 percent of the cancers in American women. Women fear it because we know that it is a silent killer, slipping into our lives quietly and unobtrusively until it is firmly rooted. Currently, 75 percent of all women diagnosed with ovarian cancer die from the disease; but when the disease is detected early, 80 percent of women are survivors at the five-year mark. Obviously, a screening test would be of great benefit to us all—if for no other reason than peace of mind—but no effective screen yet exists. Much research is underway to find an effective screen, and early indicators look as though the resultant screen will rely on DNA markers in the blood or urine.

Tests that have been considered so far are:

1. Bimanual examination is the part of your gynecological physical exam where your doctor uses two fingers in your vagina and the other hand on your abdomen, feeling inside your pelvis, as described for Frannie in chapter 3. While a standard part of every well-woman exam, it is very difficult to detect enlargement of the ovaries in any but the thinnest women. Indeed, a study done in the late 1990s, comparing the results of pelvic exams done by some of the most lauded experts with the findings on ultrasound exams, demonstrated that the best of us is only about 40 percent accurate in picking up ovarian pathology on physical exam. If this pathology is ovarian cancer, it is likely to have

spread outside the ovary by the time we are able to feel it on pelvic exam.

2. Ultrasound exam is useful in individual women, but has been disappointing as a screen of large numbers of women. There are a number of prospective randomized trials in progress to assess the usefulness of ultrasound as a screen for ovarian cancer. Currently, in practice, it is used to evaluate women who are felt to be at highest risk, which means women with strong family histories of ovarian cancer.

3. Blood tests that measure a protein called Ca125 are used in women suspected of having ovarian cancer. This may be used together with ultrasound in women at high risk, although no firm protocol exists for doing so. Ongoing studies are assessing the utility of this test as a means of screening, both alone and in combination with ultrasound. The National Cancer Institute's Prostate, Lung, Colorectal, and Ovarian (PLCO) Cancer Screening Trial is assessing the combined technique. While we eagerly and hopefully await the trial results, we strongly suggest that women at high risk have pelvic ultrasound and Ca125 tests every six months (see chapter 15).

Thyroid Disease

Although thyroid disease causes high morbidity, there is no recommendation for routine screening because there is insufficient evidence that it is useful. The exception to this is the screening for congenital hypothyroidism (low level of thyroid hormones, sometimes in association with goiter or swelling of the thyroid gland) that is done as part of the neonatal screening blood work for babies. It is imperative that newborns be diagnosed as quickly as possible if they have congenital hypothyroidism because if it is not treated soon, the baby's intelligence is adversely affected. There is no similar evidence that screening asymptomatic adults impacts future morbidity, but certainly doctors need to be sensitive to symptoms that warrant testing women for thyroid disease, such as fatigue, change in weight, memory problems, and constipation, to mention a few.

There are many other conditions for which there are no screens because no effective method exists, the condition is too uncommon to warrant testing whole populations, or because early detection would not lead to early treatment, either because no treatment exists or because early treatment does not improve the course of the illness.

15 *Genetic Screening*

Tyler is the daughter of Jean Morris's friend Kathleen, who died of breast cancer. Kathleen's mother, Sarah, also died young, but of ovarian cancer. Tyler was a teenager when her mother died and didn't realize the significance of her family history until she was going over her new patient questionnaire with a nurse practitioner at Planned Parenthood. This was the first that Tyler learned of the possibility of an inherited gene that increases the risk of both breast and ovarian cancer. She was especially dumbfounded to hear that it was more common in Ashkenazi Jews, her maternal origin. After thoughtful consideration and a long telephone chat with her dad, Tyler decided to have the genetic testing to see if she had this gene.

First of all, what is a gene? Within almost every cell of your body, there is a nucleus. Mature red blood cells are exceptions, but we are not going to talk about them because they are not relevant to this discussion. Imagine the cell is an egg, and the nucleus is the yolk. Within the nucleus are the chromosomes, which are packages of genes. In the human, each cell nucleus contains twenty-two pairs of autosomes, or nonsex chromosomes, and one pair of sex chromosomes—XX in the female and XY in the male. This is the normal situation, although abnormalities can occur. Such abnormalities may entail extra or missing chromosomes, or chromosomes that seem to have traded bits of gene material with each other.

As we've said, chromosomes are packages of genes and the genes, in turn, are composed of the basic building material of life: deoxyribonucleic acid, better known as DNA. The DNA is made up of long intertwined strands with molecules arranged in varying sequences, much like a double-strand necklace with gems repeating at different intervals. These sequences of molecules act as a code that allows the DNA to convey messages related to how particular tissues will develop, grow, and function. Within the DNA genes are matched in pairs. To determine a particular characteristic, at least one pair of genes is always involved; however, human genetics is very complex and often involves more than one pair of genes. Each person's chromosomes contain somewhere between twenty-five and thirty thousand genes, which convey all the information needed for that person to develop as a fetus in the womb, and to grow, mature, and live a life as a unique individual. Half of the genes involved in a person's development come from the father at the time of conception and the other half from the mother. Everyone gets an X chromosome from their mother and either an X or a Y chromosome from their father, which determines their sex. The contribution of half of the genes from each parent results in a random mixing of the contributed genes on the chromosomes, so that the end result is diversity. Most people are aware of the familial resemblances of siblings, but know that none are truly identical unless they are twins sharing exactly the same genetic material from their parents. A human genome is all the genetic information about a person neatly packaged into that person's chromosomes—kind of like a biologic microchip.

Along with all the information about the color of your hair, eyes, and skin—as well as whether or not you will inherit Dad's hooked nose or Mom's rosebud mouth—everyone has the possibility of having certain alterations in the genes that can predispose the development of certain diseases or conditions. We call these alterations mutations, and they may be present on either the autosomes or the X chromosomes. (Little information is carried on the Y chromosome.) You also need to realize that just as some people are forceful and domineering while others are shy and reticent, we also have genes that are dominant and those that are recessive. A dominant gene causes its coded characteristic to appear in the individual even if its paired gene carries a different characteristic—it dominates. A recessive gene needs to act in pairs—meaning that the characteristic in question has to come from both parents and be coded on both of the paired genes in order for the characteristic to appear in the person. For example, Huntington's chorea, the disease that Woody Guthrie made famous, is coded by one dominant gene; and if the person inherits that gene from his or her parent, the disease is passed on. Cystic fibrosis, on the other hand, is a disease that is carried by a recessive gene, so it needs a gene from each parent to be inherited. If a person inherits one gene for a recessive disorder, she is said to be a carrier for this trait and may pass it on to the next generation, if she mates with another carrier or someone who has the disease.

Of course, not all conditions that "run in families" are inherited through a single gene. We know, for instance, that high blood pressure and diabetes may be inherited, but in these conditions several as yet unidentified genes are responsible. And clearly it's not only the genes that are responsible for disease developing—the environment, lifestyle, and diet all play a big part. (And of course, characteristics that a parent has acquired, such as a funny shaped nose because it has been broken or a limp from having polio, are not passed on to children.)

Tyler was tested and learned that she had inherited the BRCA1 gene mutation from her mother, Kathleen. Does this mean that she has a 100 percent certainty of developing breast cancer? No . . . genes have a variable ability to make their presence felt. This is called penetrance, the varying ability of a particular gene to actually manifest itself as disease. In the case of the BRCA1 gene, it has less than a 100 percent penetrance or chance of causing cancer in the person inheriting it. In fact, it gives Tyler a 20 to 40 percent chance of developing ovarian cancer and a 40 to 80 percent chance of developing breast cancer. Obviously, when it comes to breast cancer, the gene has greater penetrance.

This is a very simple explanation. Genetics is actually quite complex, and genetic counselors are trained to understand and keep up with these complexities. Genetic testing may be done because a woman is part of a certain population group, for example Ashkenazi Jewish women, or because of a family history. In Tyler's case, both conditions were present. Any woman who knows she has a genetic risk for a particular disease or condition or is contemplating being tested for such genetic risks should receive genetic counseling. We can expect this to become increasingly important as technology becomes more sophisticated and we learn to screen for more conditions. It is unconscionable to give people cold facts without putting them in a context of possibilities.

We already screen for some chromosomal abnormalities, such as Down's syndrome. But this indicator doesn't always mean the chromosomes themselves are examined. The fetal nuchal translucency (FNT) screening is an ultrasound of the skin fold at the back of the baby's neck, done at around twelve weeks of pregnancy. It is noninvasive, and a positive result does not mean that the baby definitely has Down's syndrome—it is simply a marker for further testing. Amniocentesis is the test that actually looks at the baby's chromosomes after fluid is taken from within the uterus and is a diagnostic chromosome test. Another example of genetic screening with which many women are familiar is the heel-prick test offered to babies throughout the United States. This method is used to test for an increasing number of genetic conditions; the exact program varies from state to state. However, all states include the test for phenylketonuria, a condition that retards intellectual development if left untreated.

More and more help to available to women like Tyler, who want to know if their risk of breast or ovarian cancer is high, and if so, what they can do about it. Widespread population screening for a multitude of genetic defects is not yet implemented partially due to ethical concerns. Some high-risk populations, however, are being offered screening for particular inherited health problems. Examples include people with a family history of Huntington's disease, Tay-Sachs disease, hemochromatosis, and familial breast and ovarian cancer (like Tyler).

We have mentioned that colon cancer may have a familial basis. About 80 percent of colon cancer cases seem to occur sporadically but a sizeable proportion, around 20 percent, does run in families. So a family history of colon cancer should alert you to the need to discuss early screening with your doctor. There are two well-known genetic conditions that indicate a predisposition to colon cancer—familial adenomatous polyposis (FAP) and hereditary nonpolyposis colorectal cancer (HNPCC). These daunting terms simply mean that the first condition is associated with polyps growing on the bowel walls, whereas the second is a cancer that develops without the prior appearance of polyps. Polyps in the colon are very common and usually are not cancerous, as we explained when we told you about Jean's experiences in chapter 6. FAP is associated with large numbers of polyps that can develop even in childhood; removal of the colon (colectomy) is generally recommended for those diagnosed with the condition. A number of other less common genetic conditions also are associated with colon cancer. Women and men with a family history of colon and rectal cancer can now have genetic testing to see whether or not they are predisposed to developing these cancers, and if so, can take appropriate action—at the very least they can have regular screening tests. Women who test positive for HNPCC also have a greater risk of developing cancer of the ovary and cancer of the endometrium and may be offered the various screening tests we've described for those cancers.

Again, we must reiterate that much of this screening is for *potential* illness, not illness in the here-and-now, and often not inevitable illness. Many factors can impact the development of an actual disease or condition. Also please note that having a negative result for genetic test for a condition that runs in your family, such as breast or colon cancer, does not mean that you are completely risk free of developing that cancer. It simply reduces your chances to those of the general population, and you should continue screening with the tests recommended for the general population.

With the help of Mark, a very supportive partner, a good genetic counselor and family doctor, plus a close extended family, Tyler has developed a positive attitude toward her unwelcome genetic package. "There's a good chance I'll get both these cancers if I do nothing to prevent it; there's also a good chance that I won't, and hey, there are things I can do to help prevent cancer or to catch it early. I'm grateful for the technology that allowed me to know that I have to take care of myself, and I have learned the valuable lesson that I have to live each day fully— something that's true for all of us, but some of us are blessed by finding it out soon enough to live our lives fully." For the moment Tyler will have biannual pelvic ultrasounds and Ca 125 blood testing (as described in our chapter on ovarian cancer) as well as annual mammograms from the age of twenty-five.

In the genetic counselor's waiting room, Tyler met a woman named Anne, thirty years old, whose mother also died of breast cancer. Anne's mother was from Sweden and Anne is uncertain about the health history of other maternal relatives. Anne has not had the same support that Tyler has enjoyed: her husband, Jake, has just started his own software consulting business and is preoccupied with business matters. His approach to Anne's news that she has the BRCA1 gene is "Buck up, it might never happen." He refuses to talk about the implications in regard to the children they haven't had and how this news might impact their plan to have a baby in about three years. (The BRCA gene mutations can occur in both females and males, so Anne can pass the tendency to either a daughter or a son.) Anne feels very lonely and lost, and she has begun seeing a psychiatrist and taking antidepressant medications.

Anne's case illustrates some of the ethical issues involved in testing people for potential problems. Instead of the information being used positively, as in Tyler's case, it can cause worry, anxiety, even severe depression, and a feeling of inevitability that is frequently out of all proportion to the facts. Keep in mind that we are statistically at risk for a huge number of accidents and diseases—besides we must eventually succumb to something. As far as cancer is concerned, there is always a risk for the whole population of getting a particular cancer. For example, the overall population of women in the United States has a risk of about 1 in 11 for developing breast cancer some time in life. But most of these women will not die from breast cancer. Everyone undergoing genetic testing needs to be aware that there are possible psychological consequences for those with positive results; equally, counselors and others concerned with health care provision need to be able to recognize and treat negative reactions to such information being conveyed to a person undergoing testing. If you are contemplating testing, we first urge you to talk through all aspects of the process with a trained genetic counselor.

It also has become clear that people who find they don't carry a gene mutation known to occur in their family can nevertheless suffer psychological consequences of this knowledge. It can be devastating for one sibling to learn that she is free of a gene, but her brother (or sister) does have it. Relief may be overwhelmed by feelings of guilt, what is sometimes called "survivor guilt." Michele's patient Judy is a good example of this: Judy, in her mid-twenties, and her older brother Dennis have been tested recently for Huntington's chorea which their father, Vic, died from in his late fifties. Dennis carries the gene and will develop this slowly debilitating condition; Judy does not carry the gene. Now Judy feels guilty; why should she be so lucky when her brother isn't? And there's a little twinge of anxiety, too—maybe she's going to have to help look after Dennis; and having already nursed her father before his death, she feels guiltier for even allowing this thought to enter her head. Judy is just as much in need of help and support at this stage as Anne and Dennis.

Other concerns about genetic testing have to do with the use of the information; if you are known to have the gene for Huntington's disease, or for breast cancer, for example, how will insurers or employers treat you? Do you have a legal or ethical responsibility to give an insurance company the information? Can they, and do they, use such information to discriminate against people with positive results? These are among the many ethical concerns connected to genetic testing. Tyler has a life insurance policy, and she gets credit for the fact that she does not smoke cigarettes, which most people find reasonable. But now should she tell the company that she has an increased chance of breast and ovarian cancer before the policy matures when Tyler turns fifty-five? Why should she be discriminated against when another woman, who also has the possibility of having the gene mutation, but has not taken the test, does not face discrimination? And then there's the fact that breast cancer, as we've just mentioned, is pretty common in the general population of women. Most breast cancers occur in women who don't have the BRCA or other similar mutations. We just don't know all the factors that bring about the development of cancer. Most states have laws in place to prevent people in Tyler's position from being discriminated against if they have insurance prior to testing. Of course your medical records are supposed to be totally private, but in reality, privacy is often breached. Insurance companies may be able to access certain information if they have agreed to insure you, and in answering the company's questions before insurance is provided you have a legal obligation to inform them of any positive test results. If possible discrimination is a concern to you, discuss this with your genetic advisor before deciding to have a particular test. The National Human Genome Research Institute's website lists each state's laws on insurance and employment discrimination. (See the websites listed at the end of this chapter.)

Some further difficulties with genetic testing can be illustrated with another story from our practices. Caroline's patient Aimee was diagnosed with breast cancer three years ago, at the early age of thirty-three. She had cancer treatment, which so far seems to have been successful, as well as genetic testing that showed a gene mutation predisposing her to breast cancer. Aimee has a sister, Janey, from whom she has been estranged for many years and who lives in a distant part of the country. Aimee stubbornly refused to communicate this information to Janey, despite much discussion with Caroline and the surgeon who performed her treatment. There was no way, legally, for anyone except Aimee to advise Janey that she was at greater risk and to consider early screening herself. Six months ago, Janey was found to have breast cancer, as well. In her case, the disease was more advanced than Aimee's was at diagnosis. Although the two sisters have reconciled, if given the information earlier, Janey might have gone for breast screening sooner and had a better outcome. It is generally recommended that information be shared with family members, so that they can make their own decisions to be screened, or not. But you cannot be compelled to do this, and information about your health is confidential as far as your family is concerned. Information about common familial conditions and cancers is in table 15.1. A complete list would be enormous—and the number of genetic conditions for which testing can be done is being steadily increased. Currently there are more than two hundred labs in the United States offering more than nine hundred different tests. Although family physicians and other health care providers are well informed in general, most want to refer a woman seeking specific genetic testing to a genetic counselor for advice about her particular problem. We should note that the family physician is still the most important person for initially identifying people with a family history that might heighten their risk of developing certain cancers or other conditions. The family physician is usually the person who knows you and your family best, and is the person whose responsibility it is to refer you to a genetic counselor or cancer genetics specialist. And the link with the family physician is important in other ways. The genetics specialist may counsel various options for risk reduction, such as increased surveillance or surgical prophylaxis, and it is the family physician that helps arrange treatment.

A note about family medical history—despite the best intentions, people can be wrong about the diagnosis made of another family member. This is particularly so with cancers inside the abdomen; one very good reason is their nasty habit of spreading from one organ to another. Cancers of the breast, stomach, and uterus often spread to the ovaries, for example, and so a relative not directly involved may believe her aunt or cousin has had primary ovarian cancer. A doctor or counselor taking a family history may need information from other doctors or hospitals before an accurate assessment of a particular woman's risk can be given.

Another problem that needs to be mentioned, at least, is that no testing is completely free of possible lab error. At the moment in the United States, no regulations are in place to ensure the consistency and accuracy of genetic testing. Some companies are making tests commercially available anyway, but people need to know that some of these are unregulated and that not all labs are licensed.

In our practice, we routinely test for certain genetic disorders during pregnancy. You can ask your doctor to be checked for others that have a strong presence in your family. We have listed some of the more common DNA-based tests ordered by doctors, in addition to those already mentioned.

If you have concerns about any of these, discuss them with your doctor and consider seeing a qualified genetic counselor. Any person considering a genetic test needs to be thoroughly informed about why they are having the test, what a positive and a negative result means, whether or not results may be

Table 15.1 Common Genetic Tests

Disease/Condition	Abbreviation	Manifestations
Alpha-1-antitrytptin deficiency	AAT	Emphysema, liver disease
Amyotrophic lateral sclerosis or Lou Gehrig's disease	ALS	Loss of motor function, death
Alzheimer's disease	APOE	Late senile dementia
Ataxia telangiectasia	AT	Progressive loss of muscle control
Charcot-Marie-Tooth	CMT	Loss of feeling in limbs
Congenital adrenal hyperplasia	CAH	Adrenal hormone deficiency
Cystic fibrosis	CF	Affects lungs and pancreas
Dystonia	DYT	Muscle rigidity, twisting
Fanconi anemia	FA	Blood disease
Factor V-Leiden	FVL	Blood clotting disorder
Familial adenomatous polyposis	FAP	Colon cancer at young age
Familial breast and ovarian cancer	BRCA 1 and 2	Breast and ovarian cancer at young age
Fragile X syndrome	FRAX	Mental retardation
Gaucher's disease	GD	Bone, liver, and spleen
Hemophilia	HEMA and HEMB	Bleeding disorders
Hemochromatosis	HFE	Iron storage disorder
Huntington's disease	HD	Degenerative neurologic disorder
Myotonic dystrophy	MD	Progressive muscle weakness

(Continued)

Table 15.1 (Continued)

Disease/Condition	Abbreviation	Manifestations
Muscular dystrophy— Duchenne or Becker	DMD	Mild to severe muscle weakness
Neurofibromatosis 1	NF 1	Benign nerve tumors
Nonpolyposis colon cancer	CA	Early colon cancer
Phenylketonuria	PKU	Mental retardation due to missing enzyme
Polycystic kidney disease	APKD	Kidney failure
Prader Willi/Angelman	PW/A	Neurologic symptoms
Sickle-cell disease	SS	Blood disorder
Spinocerebellar ataxia, type 1	SCA1	Neurologic symptoms— involuntary movement, reflexes
Spinal muscular atrophy	SMA	Severe, progressive muscle wasting
Tay-Sachs disease	TS	Neurologic disorder— fatal in childhood
Thalassemias	THAL	Blood disease (anemia)

inconclusive, and what kind of follow-up may be required. You should be asked to give your consent in writing. Studies have shown that even licensed labs are not always meeting these conditions. Without strict attention to these requirements, inaccurate and potentially dangerous information (in the sense of false reassurance) may be given. Much more information is available on the website of the National Human Genome Research Institute.

Resources

INTERNET

National Human Genome Research Institute's website, www
.nhgri.nih.gov, has a wide range of information available about
genetic testing that can be done in your area. You can also consult two other websites to obtain reliable information: www
.geneclinics.org and www.nci.nih.gov, the National Cancer
Institute.

16 *Laboratory Tests*

Like many of us, Frannie is curious about the blood tests her doctor orders. She usually hears that "everything is OK," "normal," or "your cholesterol is good and you're not anemic," but no one has ever explained what the tests are and why they are done. This chapter covers the three most common types of lab tests: hematology, chemistry screens, and urinalysis, as well as more particularly targeted tests and diagnostic tests. Charts of normal results are included as reference guidelines. (Keep in mind that values can vary somewhat from one lab to another.)

All hematology and chemistry tests are blood tests, and obviously, there must be a mechanism for getting your blood to test. This is called venipuncture and involves drawing blood from your vein into a vacuum tube by means of a needle puncture into the vein. The vein most commonly used is the one in the crook of your elbow—we call it the antecubital vein. If you are heavy, have scarring in this area, or if the vein is difficult to access for other reasons, the next most common choice is the largest vein on the back of your hand. The technician drawing the blood first disinfects the skin over the vein, then slips a needle, bevel side up, into the vein, and attaches the vacutainer tube into which the blood flows (or more accurately, is sucked by the vacuum in the tube). The bevel is up so that blood will not leak around the bottom of the needle, cause a mess, and increase the possibility of bruising afterward. Venipuncture usually doesn't hurt beyond a pinprick; the skin area over the antecubital vein isn't terribly sensitive, and if your vein is easily accessed, the whole procedure takes only a few minutes. You can help make the procedure easy by taking care to be well hydrated and warm. Drink a glass or two of water prior to your appointment and do everything possible to make sure your skin is warm. If you have a history of difficult blood draws and know your hand will be used, wrap a hot pack around the hand or hold it under warm, running water until it is warm enough to redden the skin. This warming process dilates your veins and makes them more prominent.

Now that the blood is in the tube and at the lab, we can talk more about these particular tests and what they tell us. We group them by physiological categories, just as your doctor does.

Hematology

First, let us consider the hematology report. This entire grouping of tests is known as the CBC or complete blood count. (In some parts of the world it is called the whole blood count, but it has the same meaning.) The hematology report is a common screening test. We first look at the white blood count (WBC). If elevated, we order a white cell differential, or a breakdown of the various types of white cells counted. Many automated CBCs report this routinely. Tuck this in your mind, while we explain the rest of the CBC.

The hemoglobin (Hgb), hematocrit (Hct), and the red cell count tell us about how much hemoglobin you have and the number of red cells carrying that hemoglobin. The hemoglobin is the oxygen-carrying component of red cells. Hematocrit is the volume of the packed red blood cells in a very small glass tube (capillary tube) measured after the tube full of blood has been centrifuged, packing the red cells together. In the simplest scenario, all of these may be low and we can readily say that you are anemic. If so, we then go on to do other types of tests to tell us why. Anemia involves one or more of these values being low; in

Table 16.1 Hematology

Test	Normal Range
White blood cells (x 1,000)	4.8–10.8
Red blood cells (x 1,000,000)	4.2–5.4
Hemoglobin (g/dL)	12–16
Hematocrit %	37–47
MCV (cubic micrometers)	81–99
MCH (mmg)	28–32
MCHC %	32–26
Platelets (x 1,000)	140–440
Reticulocytes %	0.5–1.5
ESR (Westergren) (sed rate)	
Under 50 yrs old	0–20
Over 50 yrs old	0–30

Note: All values are for women.

the case of B_{12} or folate deficiency anemia, there is also an increased MCV, or volume of the red cell.

An elevation of the number of red cells, hemoglobin, and/or hematocrit may mean a number of things. This happens physiologically at high altitudes when your body has to accommodate for decreased oxygen availability. There are other conditions, both benign and not, in which there is an increase in red cells or hemoglobin or both. Hemochromatosis is one of the most common genetic disorders; it is an iron storage disease, often first suspected when a doctor notices that someone's hemoglobin is unusually high. There are disorders of the blood-making mechanisms of the body in which unusually high numbers of red cells are produced. In all of these cases, elevated red cell count, hemoglobin, and hematocrit are the first clues that further investigations need to be done.

As we've mentioned, MCV is the mean red cell volume, and when it is larger than normal, leads us to check for vitamin B_{12} or folic acid deficiency. MCHC is the mean red cell hemoglobin and if it is lower than normal, it is a clue that there is an iron deficiency. In these cases, we draw further bloods to test for serum B_{12} and folic acid levels or for serum iron levels and what we call total iron binding capacity—or, in other words, how many parking places for iron on the red cell hemoglobin are already occupied. Obviously, if there are many parking spots left, there is a need for more iron.

The reticulocyte count is important if a person is anemic or has lost blood because it is a count of less mature red cells, and clearly, there is an increase when there is an increase in production in response to need. Seeing reticulocytes in an anemic person is reassuring, because it is a sign of red cell production.

Platelets are strange little fragments of cells that are very important in our ability to clot our blood. Decreased or elevated platelet counts have many meanings, but the initial finding is a signal that we need to look for certain infectious diseases, blood diseases, or malignancies. The clinical picture helps us to decide which we are looking for in a particular instance. A very small increase or decrease may simply lead us to repeat the test.

The ethrythrocyte sedimentation rate (ESR) is a nonspecific test that we use as an indicator of active disease, be it infectious, inflammatory, or malignant. The result shows how elevated it is and can offer a hint into which category the illness may fall, but tells little else. For example, when people complain of achy joints, it is commonly used to get a fairly quick (one hour) idea of whether or not an active inflammatory arthritis is present.

Chemistries

A routine chemistry screen shows the many substances transported in the blood outside the red and white blood cells. Many of these are attached to proteins that are a normal component of

Table 16.2 Chemistries

Test	Normal Range
Albumin	3.4–5.0 g/dL
Alkaline phosphatase	50–136 U/L
Amylase	25–125 U/L
Bilirubin, total	0–1.0 mg/dL
Blood urea nitrogen (BUN)	7–18 mg/dL
Calcium	8.5–11.5 mg/dL
Cholesterol	0–200 mg/dL
Chloride	101–111 mEq/L
CPK	21–232 U/L
CO_2	21–32 mEq/L
Creatinine	0.6–1.0 (women)
Gamma GT	15–85 IU/L
Glucose	70–110 mg/dL
HDL (high-density lipoprotein)	39–96 mg/dL (women)
LDH (lactic dehydrogenase)	100–190 IU/L
Magnesium	1.8–2.5 mg/dL
Phosphorus	2.5–4.9 mg/dL
Potassium	3.6–5.2 mEq/L
SGOT (AST)	15–37 IU/L
SGPT (ALT)	30–65 IU/L
Sodium	135–145 mEq/L
Total protein	6.4–8.2 g/dL
Triglycerides	30–200 mg/dL
Uric acid	2.6–7.2 mg/dL

the serum in which the red blood cells are suspended. In reading a chemistry report, we quickly scan for any abnormal readings and then see if any related values are abnormal. For example, if the glucose is elevated, indicating possible diabetes, we also check to see that the serum potassium is OK and that the electrolytes (sodium, potassium, chloride, and CO_2) are normal. Now, let's look through the chemistries.

- Albumin is one of the protein components in the blood and is an indicator of liver function and nutritional status. It is grouped with other liver function tests.
- Alkaline phosphatase is a blood enzyme that is an indicator of liver function and bone metabolism. It is included in liver function tests.
- Amylase is not part of a routine chemistry screen, but is ordered if you have severe abdominal pain. It is elevated in pancreatitis, or inflammation of the pancreas. When pancreatitis is suspected, another pancreatic enzyme, lipase, is also measured.
- Total bilirubin is a measure of the bilirubin group of pigments produced by the liver. An elevated bilirubin can indicate liver disease or excessive breakdown of red blood cells. Once in a while, a person will have a persistent slight elevation of their bilirubin as a result of a genetic enzyme defect; these are not usually disease states, but need to be differentiated from other causes of elevated bilirubin.
- BUN or blood urea nitrogen is an indicator of the breakdown of protein in the body and how well the kidney is handling it. This is an indicator of kidney function.
- Calcium is one of the body minerals. Abnormalities in the serum calcium do not commonly reflect dietary intake, but may reflect problems with the parathyroid glands (four little glands in your neck), Vitamin D metabolism, kidney disease, some bone diseases, some cancers, and malnutrition or

malabsorption. If there is an abnormal result in an otherwise healthy person, the test is simply repeated because technical problems, such as a tourniquet that's too tight, can alter the results.

- Cholesterol is a familiar term to most people today. In fact, one can overhear incredibly boring conversations in restaurants in which parties of diners may be playing the cholesterol one-upmanship game: "Yes, my last cholesterol was more than 300 and I have to take XYZ medicine every day." "Oh, my dear, that's nothing, mine was more than 400 until I went on the latest, most advertised potion of the day!" Facetiousness aside, most people are well aware that cholesterol is one of the body fats. Some of the measured cholesterol is actually manufactured by our body and the rest reflects our diet. Cholesterol is one of the blood lipids, and we often refer to a lipid profile.

- Chloride is one of the body's electrolytes or salts. We usually look at all salts as a group; they may be altered in disease states, such as vomiting and diarrhea, lung disease, and metabolic diseases like diabetes.

- CPK is more commonly called CK, or creatine kinase, today. This is an enzyme that can reflect problems with muscle. There are subtests that can narrow this further to heart muscle versus skeletal muscle.

- CO_2 or carbon dioxide is another of the blood electrolytes and is most commonly disturbed in chronic lung disease.

- Creatinine is an indicator of metabolic waste products that have been processed by the kidney as well as a marker of kidney function. Creatinine and the BUN are looked at together.

- Gamma GT is one of the liver enzymes and is commonly elevated in liver diseases especially hepatitis. It is one of the "liver function tests."

- Glucose, or blood sugar, is another commonly known test. This test is used to screen for diabetes mellitus (sweet water) and to monitor the disease. Because of the prevalence and implications of diabetes and prediabetic conditions, this is a routine screening test.

- HDL is commonly known as the "good cholesterol." The letters stand for high-density lipoprotein. In this case more is better, and a high HDL is good. Some people may note that LDL, or low-density lipoprotein, is not listed. This is because it is most commonly a derived value, meaning it is calculated by subtracting the HDL from the total cholesterol. In cases in which the blood lipids (these are both part of that category) are very high, we can send a blood sample to a reference laboratory to have a "direct LDL" or true LDL measured.

- Magnesium is one of the blood salts, and until recent years its importance was underestimated. Magnesium is critical to the proper functioning of muscle, including heart muscle, nerves, and many others affected by these. To get a truly accurate measurement of your magnesium status, your doctor may have to order a measurement in both the plasma and the red cells, because there is a constant equilibrium of magnesium between them.

- Phosphorus is another of the blood minerals; abnormalities in phosphorus may occur in kidney disease, parathyroid disease, malnutrition, malabsorption, and Vitamin D deficiency.

- Potassium is one of the blood salts and is included in electrolyte profiles. It is abnormal in conditions affecting the acidity of the blood (diabetic ketoacidosis), kidney disease, diseases of the adrenal glands, diarrhea and vomiting, and sometimes from too aggressive medical treatment with diuretics (or, unfortunately, when people with eating disorders abuse diuretics).

- Sodium is another of the blood electrolytes and can be abnormal in certain hormonal disorders (adrenal or pituitary glands), kidney, liver, or heart disease, vomiting or diarrhea, dehydration, and iatrogenic causes, such as too aggressive IV fluid therapy or diuretics.

- Total protein represents the total albumin and globulin in the blood. The globulin fraction is simply a subtraction of the albumin from the total protein. Certain cancers, liver or kidney disease, chronic infection or inflammation, and malabsorption or malnutrition can affect the total protein.

- Triglycerides are another of the lipids or body fats. Triglycerides are indicative of the total calorie content of your diet and not just fat intake. High triglycerides can be suspicious of future diabetes and are commonly elevated in diabetics.

- Uric acid is elevated in gout, kidney failure, some cancers, and in tissue destruction. There are some uncommon congenital diseases in which you see low uric acid values. The significance in these cases is not known. In gout, crystals of uric acid can be recovered from aspirated fluid from gouty joints.

Urinalysis

Our kidneys do a remarkable job of which we are mostly unaware. Day and night they work away to maintain important substances in our blood, such as salts, at just the right levels. They also filter out waste products and help to keep us well hydrated. A number of different chemicals are excreted through the kidneys, in good and bad health, and measuring these substances in the urine can be helpful in making a diagnosis of specific complaints.

- Specific gravity reflects our ability to concentrate our urine. We all know that our first urine of the day is darker than it is later in the day after we've had plenty to drink. This is because that first urine is concentrated.

Table 16.3 Urinalysis

Test	Normal Range or Value
Specific gravity	1.005–1.030
pH	4.5–8.0
Urobilinogen	0.1–1.0 EU/dL
Blood	Negative
Bilirubin	Negative
Ketones	Negative
Glucose	Negative
Protein	Negative
Leukocytes (white blood cells)	Negative
Nitrites	Negative
HCG (pregnancy test)	Negative (unless you want to be)

The inability to concentrate can reflect either pituitary or kidney disease.

- PH reflects the acidity of the urine and is a partial reflection of the body's several very elegant mechanisms to ensure that the body fluids are maintained at exactly the right equilibrium between acidity and alkalinity. These are called buffering systems.

- Urobilinogen reflects the excretion of some of the bile salts made by the liver.

- Blood is, of course, a sign of bleeding somewhere in the urinary tract—kidneys, ureters, or most commonly, the bladder. This can be a sign of infection, inflammation, a stone, or tumor.

- Bilirubin is, as previously mentioned, one of the bile pigments, or salts, made in the liver. It is not normally found in the urine, but can be a sign of liver or gall bladder disease.

- Ketones are a byproduct of protein breakdown and are present when body proteins (muscles) are metabolized, such as in starvation or abnormal metabolic states like diabetes.
- Glucose is normally absent from the urine, but may be present in diabetes or in kidney disease, or sometimes, in people whose kidneys normally spill glucose at a lower blood level than the usual 180 mg/dL.
- Protein in urine can indicate infection, inflammation, kidney disease, or occasionally a benign condition.
- Leukocytes or white blood cells in urine usually are associated with infection, but in women it also may be from a vaginal discharge. We keep this in mind when we look at urinalysis results.
- Nitrites in urine are indicative of a urinary infection.
- Human choriogonadotrophic (HCG) hormone is, of course, the basis of the pregnancy test that many of us have done at home. In this case, the looked for result depends on your desire to be pregnant or not.

This covers screening tests that are commonly done when you go to your doctor for a routine physical. There are other common tests that are generated by particular symptoms. Some of them follow.

Thyroid Tests

Thyroid disease is very common among women, especially as they become a little more mature. The most common version of thyroid disease in women is autoimmune thyroiditis (Hashimoto's thyroiditis), which tends to run in a family's female line. Although this is common, experts have ruled that there is insufficient evidence that screening provides enough benefit to justify routine screening for thyroid disease. Nevertheless, many doctors working with women test them at least once after the age of forty.

- TSH is the thyroid-stimulating hormone secreted by the pituitary gland. This hormone level is elevated when there is a decrease in the thyroid's ability to put out thyroid hormone (T_4 and T_3). You can think of TSH as a supervisor putting out increased effort to make the underperforming employees under his control work harder. The normal range of TSH levels is 0.4 to 5.5.
- We usually test for T_4, the active form of thyroid hormone. T_3 is T_4 minus an iodine molecule and is less often responsible for thyroid disease. In hyperthyroidism, too much thyroid hormone is produced and the TSH value is low.
- Antimicrosomal antibodies are made by your body and directed against your thyroid gland. They are virtually always present in Hashimoto's thyroiditis and 80 percent present in Graves disease.

Autoimmune Diseases

Autoimmune conditions occur because the body manufactures antibodies to certain of its own tissues; these antibodies then treat the tissues as "foreign" and attack them, causing chronic damage. Comprised of a large group of diseases, it is beyond the scope of this book to cover all of the laboratory tests that may be involved in diagnosing them. Thus, only the more prevalent ones are included.

- The ESR or sedimentation rate has long been a mainstay in testing, but is gradually being replaced by the C-reactive protein, which is more specific for inflammation. C-reactive protein is elevated when there is inflammation. A negative result is normal.
- ANA or antinuclear antibody test looks for antibodies made by your body against the nuclei of your own cells. This may be elevated in lupus and sometimes in other autoimmune

diseases, such as scleroderma, Sjogren's syndrome, poly-myositis, and some types of chronic hepatitis. The normal result is negative or less than 1:40. Certain drugs can cause false positive ANA results.

- RF or rheumatoid factor is another antibody that may be present in people with rheumatoid arthritis. A negative rheumatoid factor doesn't necessarily rule out rheumatoid arthritis. RF may be present in joint aspirates as well as the blood.
- Anti-DNA antibody is sometimes found in lupus, but not in other autoimmune diseases. When present, it also can be used to monitor the success of treatment.
- Anti–smooth muscle antibody may be present in some types of chronic active hepatitis and may help your doctor with diagnosis.
- Antimitochondrial antibody is present in primary biliary cirrhosis and often helps in the diagnosis of this disease.
- Antiphospholipid antibodies may be found in lupus. This antibody is associated with blood clots within blood vessels, habitual miscarriage, and certain neurological disorders.
- HLA or human lymphocyte antigen typing may be done to help diagnose diseases strongly associated with HLA sub-types, such as the association of HLA-B27 with anklyosing spondylitis.
- The term serum complement refers to a group of proteins in the blood that mediate inflammatory reactions. The serum complement screen is a blood test that measures to-tal complement and usually C_3 and C_4. The normal range for total complement is 40 to100 units. C_3 is normally 1600 micrograms/ml, and a deficiency correlates with in-creased susceptibility to infection. C_4 normally measures 600 micrograms/ml and a deficiency correlates with lupus. Complement testing is very helpful in evaluating arthritic diseases.

Diabetes

A number of tests are used to monitor diabetes. It is also important to realize that timing in relation to food intake must be considered. HgbA$_1$C is a test that allows us to have an idea of diabetic control over time, rather than simply at that particular moment. It is usually done about every three months, although in the case of a diabetic with poor glucose control, a HgbA$_1$C can be done again anytime after a twenty-eight-day interval to assess the effect of another intervention—adding insulin to an oral drug regimen for example.

HgbA$_1$C is normally 4.4 to 6.3 percent in a nondiabetic person. In a diabetic, HgbA$_1$C of 5.8 to 6 percent is excellent control and 6 to 7 percent is good control, indicating effective treatment. Results of 7.1 to 8 percent (fair control) or over 8 percent (poor control) indicates need for further treatment. It has been shown that a reduction of 1 percentage point can reduce the risk of vascular, renal, or neurological complications of diabetes by about 30 percent.

In a pregnant woman, an initial screen for blood sugar is done, with normal results being between 70 and 110 mg/dL. If this is elevated or if the woman is at high risk for diabetes (is an American Indian or has had gestational diabetes in a previous pregnancy), a one-hour glucose tolerance test may be done in early pregnancy. This test entails drinking 50 gm of a very sweet liquid (Glucola) and one hour later drawing a blood sample and analyzing it for glucose. A normal result is less than 130 mg/dL. This test is usually done routinely later in pregnancy.

Another important test in diabetes is a urine test; each time a diabetic patient is seen in clinic, her urine is tested for protein (a sign of diabetic kidney disease). If the urine is negative for protein, it is tested once yearly for micro albumin, a minute amount of protein that allows us to recognize very early kidney disease and try to intervene so that it doesn't get worse.

Many more laboratory tests are done in response to specific clinical situations. Do not feel inhibited about asking your doctor to explain any recommended tests. You'll feel less anxious if you understand what is going on and feel that you are an active partner in your care.

17 The Positive Side of Prevention

In all of our previous chapters, we've talked mostly about early detection of disease or the increased potential for disease. This is bound to leave a negative feeling, even though our intention—and the ultimate intention of these tests—is to help you prolong a good quality of life.

In this chapter we discuss those things that you can do—and over which you have control—to make your life healthier.

Many people do not eat well. Oh yes, in our society most people have adequate calorie intake, but much of it is composed of "empty" calories. This is the "junk" food that we consume in huge amounts along with sweet drinks—pop, soda, soft drinks, whatever you call them—all of which appeal to taste and texture, but supply very few vital nutrients. It is unconscionable that athletic stars endorse such foods when they must follow a healthier diet themselves to keep their bodies at peak performance capacity.

We like to keep our recommendations simple and easy to apply in daily life. One of the simplest ways we can characterize a healthy diet is to say choose foods that are close to the original form in which they grew: fresh fruits and vegetables (frozen or canned is OK if fresh is not available), whole grains, and freshly cooked meat, fish, fowl, or eggs. You know that foods in these forms are nutrient rich. Both for good health and for the esthetic of a trim body, it is best to eat between five and ten servings of fruits and vegetables each day. Another simple approach is to be sure that your serving plate is full of color, because the richly colored fruits and vegetables tend to be those that are full of nutrients like antioxidants and polyphenols that we now know are helpful in preventing many types of illness.

Avoid having a lot of fat in your diet, especially fat of animal origin. Having said that, using a little butter is better than using margarine because margarine contains some bad actors called trans fatty acids. You can make a mixture that we call "better butter" by blending one stick of butter with one-third cup of an oil such as light olive oil or canola.

There is also a need for the so-called "good fatty acids" in your diet. These are found in fish, especially sardines, salmon, tuna, bluefish, mackerel, and herring, as well as in flax seeds. A recent article in a medical journal suggested that in the future we might be testing people for the level of Omega-3 fatty acids in their blood in order to ascertain their risk of heart disease. That is in the future; the need for these fatty acids is known now.

Some doctors are advising their patients to supplement calcium in their diets because there is evidence that this may help prevent colon cancer, as well as contribute to healthy bones.

It also has been shown that taking a multiple vitamin every day contributes to general good health. So, why not? Take one that contains folate, which is one of the B vitamins—this is helpful for heart health, and also is recommended for women thinking of, or trying to, become pregnant.

Let us not ignore the huge benefit of not smoking both to you and to the people with whom you share living space. If you do smoke, quitting just may be the single most important thing you can do to reduce your risk of future illness.

Exercise is in vogue and receives a lot of press today. All health experts agree that increasing your daily exercise is important to good health. What no expert says is that you need to spend a lot of money doing this: exercise requires nothing more than the body you were born with and a desire to use it. If you enjoy going to a gym, skiing, playing squash, or participating in any such activities, please indulge yourself—these are good exercise.

However, if you don't enjoy these sports, don't think that you can't be fit. You can walk, dance, climb stairs, work in your garden, or increase your exercise in many other similar ways. Just be consistent and move more.

When you implement these suggestions, you are decreasing your risk of disease; but there are more things you can do. Skin cancer is increasing, and although there are no formal screening guidelines, it makes sense to ask your doctor to check your skin once a year, especially if you are fair-skinned. Sunscreens, hats, and sunglasses are also protections that are readily available and easy to use.

Dental health is important to overall good health; in fact, some studies point to possible connections between gum disease and heart disease. A visit to the dentist at least once yearly may save you a lot of grief down the line. Poor teeth are a major cause of poor nutrition in the elderly.

And don't neglect your feet—especially if you have any illness that affects the circulation in your feet. Diabetes and peripheral vascular disease are good examples of these. Podiatrists are professionals who are trained in the care of feet; and if you have any questions about the health or comfort of your feet, visiting a podiatrist may benefit you. It is also smart to make sure that your shoes fit well and give your feet adequate support. High heels and long pointed toes have damaged the feet of generations of women.

Happy people keep better health than those who are depressed, angry, or otherwise at odds with themselves. If you are having problems with anxiety, a sustained low mood, anger directed either at yourself or others, or thoughts that are troubling to you, seek the help of a mental health professional. People who have a connection with society outside of their own home also have healthier old ages; this does not mean that you have to have an involved career or jump into politics or anything like that, but it does mean that friendships and relationships with other people are important to us for mental and emotional well being.

Table 17.1 Recommended Immunization Schedule

Vaccine	Schedule
Tetanus/diphtheria	1 booster dose every 10 yrs.
Influenza	1 dose every yr.
Pneumococcal	1 dose for people with medical reasons.[a] After age 65, 1 dose for unvaccinated people and those vaccinated more than 5 yrs. previously
Hepatitis B	3 doses for people who have medical or other indications[b]
Hepatitis A	2 doses for people who have medical or other indications[c]
Measles, mumps, rubella	1 dose if not immunized previously or 2 doses for certain[d]
Varicella	2 doses for people who are susceptible[e]
Meningococcal	1 dose for people who have medical or other reasons[f]

a. Medical indications are chronic medical conditions such as diabetes, liver disease, kidney disease, heart disease, or any diseases requiring immunosuppressive therapy or corticosteroids. Geographic indications may be residents of Alaska Native or American Indian reservations or residents of nursing homes or other long-term care facilities.

b. Medical indications are for people who need to receive blood products; occupational indications for people involved in health and public safety and anyone involved in training. Behavioral indications apply to injecting drug users, persons with multiple sex partners in the last six months, persons with a recent diagnosis of an STD, and men who have sex with other men. Other indications are people who have sexual and/or household contact with persons who have chronic hepatitis B or HIV, patients and staff of institutions for the developmentally disabled, inmates of correctional institutions, and people who travel in countries with a high prevalence of hepatitis B.

c. Medical indications are for people with blood-clotting disorders or with liver disease. Social indications are for drug users and men who have sex with men. Occupational indications are for people who work with hepatitis A–infected animals or in research labs working with HAV. It also is recommended for people traveling in high endemic areas.

d. Adults born after 1957 should have had at least one dose of MMR unless they have reliable documentation that they have had the illnesses. A second dose is

Immunizations are important to adults, as well as children. Table 17.1 shows the recommended schedule for adult immunizations. The Advisory Committee on Immunization Practices approves this schedule. If your doctor has not suggested these immunizations to you, ask about them. They are important.

How about all the information available on the Internet? How do you know what information you can trust? We all know that there are true gems of information available as well as a lot of lumps of coal. We have provided you with websites in each of the Resources sections that we are confident contain relevant and accurate information.

Things to look when evaluating health information on a website include:

1. Who posts the site? Is it a recognized health-related institution or agency?
2. If it is an individual, are their credentials posted and can they be verified easily?
3. Are the articles authored by the individuals or agencies posting the site? If not, is the author named, and are you given that person's credentials?
4. Can you verify the facts or figures given on the site?
5. Has the website been updated recently? Can you tell if the contents are up-to-date? If there is no way to tell how long the information has been there, is it still relevant?

---

recommended for 1) people recently exposed to measles or during an outbreak, 2) people previously vaccinated with killed virus vaccine, 3) people vaccinated with unknown vaccine between 1963 and 1967, 4) students at postsecondary institutions, 5) health care workers, and 6) international travelers.

e. Recommended for all people who do not have reliable documentation of illness or a positive diagnosis of previous illness based on a blood test. Also recommended for health care workers and family contacts of immunocompromised people and those who live or work in environments where transmission of illness is facilitated. Contraindicated in pregnant women.

f. Recommended for people with certain blood diseases and for people traveling to countries with a high prevalence of illness.

6. Does the owner of the site have a commercial motive for offering you this information?

Being healthy allows us to enjoy our lives. Poor health is a serious detriment to the enjoyment of life, love, and the fulfillment of dreams. We hope that this book helps you take control of your own health and care for yourself to the best of your ability.

Resources

INTERNET

Knowing the answers to these questions will help you to have a better idea which of the vast number of health-related sites is reliable. The U.S. Department of Health and Human Services offers a service called Healthfinder, a search engine that seeks health information on the Web at *www.healthfinder.gov*. Michele has had a website called *www.askyourfamilydoc.com* since 1999, and always carefully researches the information she includes. WebMD, *www.webmd.com*, provides comprehensive medical resources for consumers and health professionals and is a highly utilized site. Most of its articles are attributed to physicians from the Cleveland Clinic. There are associated sites such as WebMD—Women's Health; WebMD—Breast Cancer; WebMD—Heart Disease; and WebMD—Weight Loss particularly aimed at those with Type 2 diabetes.

BOOKS

Of course many books are available, as well. Check our suggestions at the end of chapter 1, as well as the three well-known health encyclopedias, all recently updated, we recommend in the Further Reading section.

Appendix A
Patient Questionnaire

Name
DOB   Today's date
What is your reason for today's visit?

In the past, have you ever had any of these problems? Circle yes or no, and give the year for any yes answers.

Heart disease	Y	N	Seizures	Y	N
High blood pressure	Y	N	Kidney disease	Y	N
Pneumonia	Y	N	Migraine	Y	N
Asthma	Y	N	Joint disease	Y	N
Serious infection	Y	N	Lung disease	Y	N
Emotional problem	Y	N	Endocrine disease	Y	N

Menstrual History

Age at first period?   How many days between periods?
How many days do you bleed?   Have you been pregnant?   Y   N
How many pregnancies?   How many live births?
How many abortions?   How many miscarriages?
How many premature babies?
How many babies of ten pounds or more at birth?
Have you gone through menopause?   Y   N
If yes, at what age?
Any bleeding or spotting?   Y   N   Are you sexually active?   Y   N
With men?   Y   N   With women?   Y   N
With both?   Y   N   Do you use condoms?   Y   N
What is your birth control method?   Are you satisfied with it?   Y   N
If not, why?

Social History

Do you smoke	Y	N	If yes, how many cigarettes per day?
Do you drink alcohol?	Y	N	If yes, how much per day?
Do you take prescription medications?	Y	N	

If yes, list them on the back of this paper.

Do you take vitamins or supplements?	Y	N

If yes, list them on the back of this paper.

Do you use any drugs or medicines that are not prescribed for you?   Y   N
If yes, list them on the back of this paper.

Do you drink soda or pop?   Y   N   If yes, how many per day?
How often do you exercise?   How?
What is your job?   Do you like it?   Y   N
Are there any major stresses at home?   Y   N   If yes, please list.
Do you have relationship stress?   Y   N
Financial stress?   Y   N
Do you have animals?   Y   N   If yes, please list.
Have you traveled overseas?   Y   N   If yes, where?
When?
Have you been exposed to any environmental toxins?   Y   N
If yes, what, when, and where?
Do you wear seat belts?   Y   N
Do you have loaded guns in the house?   Y   N
Do you have difficulty walking?   Y   N

Review of Systems

Do you awaken refreshed?	Y	N	Diarrhea?	Y	N
Do you get up at night to pee?	Y	N	Have skin rashes?	Y	N
Urinate too frequently?	Y	N	Dizziness?	Y	N
Have headaches?	Y	N	Visual problems?	Y	N
Balance problems?	Y	N	Wear glasses?	Y	N
Eye pain?	Y	N	Nasal congestion?	Y	N
Hearing problems?	Y	N	Sneeze a lot?	Y	N
Sinus pressure?	Y	N	Snore?	Y	N
Runny nose?	Y	N	Memory problems?	Y	N
Fatigue easily?	Y	N	Shortness of breath?	Y	N
Chest pain?	Y	N	Cough up blood?	Y	N
Cough?	Y	N	Air hunger?	Y	N
Wheeze?	Y	N	Constipation?	Y	N
Abdominal pain?	Y	N	Painful gas?	Y	N

Vomit blood?	Y	N	Blood in stools?	Y	N
Blood in urine?	Y	N	Abnormal vaginal discharge?	Y	N

Family History

Have any of your close relatives had any of the following? Circle yes or no.
Please write relationship in the blank space provided.

Heart disease?	Y	N	Diabetes?	Y	N
Allergy?	Y	N	Obesity?	Y	N
Mental illness?	Y	N	Thyroid disease?	Y	N
Arthritis?	Y	N	Stroke?	Y	N
Immune disorder?	Y	N	Bleeding disorder?	Y	N
Alcoholism?	Y	N	Migraine?	Y	N
Cancer?	Y	N	TB?	Y	N
Kidney disease?	Y	N	Asthma?	Y	N

Please explain any yes answers:

Appendix B
Basic Screening Tests by Age

Test	19–39 years	40–50 years	50–65 years	>65 years
Blood pressure	Every 2 yrs	2 yrs*	2 yrs*	2 yrs*
Height and weight	Yearly	Yearly	Yearly	Yearly
Pap smear	1–3 yrs	1–3 yrs	1–3 yrs	1–3 yrs**
Rubella	Once			
Chlamydia	1–3 yrs	If indicated by history	If indicated by history	If indicated by history
Mammogram	If indicated by family history	2–3 yrs	Yearly	Yearly
Lipid profile	5 yrs	5 yrs	5 yrs	5 yrs
Diabetes screen		3 yrs	3 yrs	3 yrs
TSH		Once		
Colon cancer screen		FOBT yearly	See choices	See choices
Eye exam		2 yrs	2 yrs	Yearly
Bone density			3 yrs	

Source: Compiled from the recommendations of relevant national bodies.
Note: Blanks indicate no routine screening necessary.
*Unless the person is hypertensive, in which case, more often.
**May be discontinued after three previous normal Pap smears.

A Quick Guide to Terms Used in This Book

alpha fetoprotein (AFP) a chemical substance produced during pregnancy. High or low levels of AFP may point to certain abnormalities in the pregnancy.

amniocentesis a procedure in which fluid is taken from around a baby within the womb for the purpose of diagnosing certain conditions in the baby.

anemia a condition in which the hemoglobin, the oxygen-carrying pigment of the blood, is either deficient or defective.

anesthetic a drug administered either locally (on or injected into the skin, eyes, gums, or other surfaces) or generally (inhaled or intravenous), to prevent pain during surgery or other medical procedures.

angiography an X-ray technique used to outline blood vessels by administrating dyes labeled with radioactive substances that can be seen on an X-ray screen.

antioxidant a chemical present in foods or supplements that prevents oxidation in the body. Oxidation is linked to chronic diseases. Vitamin C is an example of an antioxidant.

anus the opening from the lower bowel onto the skin.

arthritis inflammation of one or more joints of the body, which can originate from one of several causes.

Ashkenazi Jew a Jewish person of Eastern European origin.

aspirated fluid fluid drawn off by needle from some part of the body, usually for diagnosic purposes.

autoimmune conditions occurring because the body develops antibodies to certain of its own tissues.

biopsy   removal of a small piece of tissue from some part of the body for microscopic examination, with the aim of making a definite diagnosis.

body mass index (BMI)   a measure of weight in relation to height that classifies a person's weight as normal, obese, or underweight; the ratio of the person's weight in kilograms divided by the square of their height in meters.

buffering   allowing a balance to be achieved between acidity and alkalinity.

carcinogens   substances predisposing an organism to the development of cancer.

centrifuge   a machine that uses very rapid rotation to separate out the constituent parts of a fluid, such as blood.

cervix   the "neck" or lower part of the uterus (womb).

chorionic gonadotrophin   a hormone produced by the placenta.

chorionic villi   part of the normal developing placenta.

colon   the lower bowel that extends from the area of appendix to the rectum and anus.

colposcopy   examination of the cervix with a telescope, usually done following an abnormal Pap smear.

congenital   present from birth. Congenital anomalies are abnormalities a baby is born with.

corticosteroid   hormones secreted by the adrenal glands; also, the group of synthetic drugs, including cortisone and prednisone, that mimic some of the actions of natural adrenal hormones.

C-reactive protein   a substance produced by inflammation anywhere in the body; testing for its presence is useful in the detection of heart disease.

CT   an X-ray technique in which a series of images are taken of "slices" of the region being examined and computer analysis constructs a three-dimensional image of that particular region or organ.

culture   the growth of organisms such as bacteria or viruses to determine the cause of an infectious illness.

cytotechnologist   a person trained to look at cells for abnormalities that may indicate cancer or precancer.

digital mammography   a technique used to convert conventional mammograms into digital photos. This is very similar to having your own conventional vacation photos put on disc or otherwise converted to digital.

deoxyribonucleic acid (DNA)   the "building blocks" of all human and animal tissue.

diuretics   drugs that promote the production of urine by the kidneys.

Doppler   a simple hand-held instrument that uses sound waves to detect blood flow, as in the heart of a fetus or in the veins and arteries of your limbs and neck.

Down's syndrome   a chromosomal abnormality with distinct physical changes and retarded intellectual capacity.

dual energy X-ray absorptiometry (DXA)   a form of low dose X-ray used to measure bone density.

dysplasia   a precancerous change in a body tissue.

electrocardiogram, electrocardiograph (EKG)   a machine used to record the normal electrical activity of the heart and the printout from the machine.

embolism   damage to organs caused by blood clots traveling in the bloodstream from other parts of the body.

endometrium   the tissue lining the uterus (womb).

endoscopy   examination of cavities within the body with specially designed telescopes; for example, colonoscopy, sigmoidoscopy.

enzymes   chemicals that help biochemical reactions to occur, for example, lipase is an enzyme that helps in the digestion of fat.

equilibrium   balance.

Food and Drug Administration (FDA)   a regulatory arm of the federal government.

fracture   a break in a bone, which may or may not result in displacement of the bone.

gestational diabetes   diabetes occurring during a pregnancy.

gynecologist   a doctor specializing in diseases and conditions of the female reproductive system.

hemoglobin A_1C   a blood pigment, the levels of which are used to assess diabetes and diabetic control.

hemorrhoids   prolapsed veins around the anus.

homocysteine   a protein that is measured to give an indication of future heart disease.

human papilloma virus (HPV)   also called wart virus, it is the cause of all warts in humans. The virus also is often present on the skin without causing warts.

iatrogenic   inadvertently caused by the actions of a doctor or some other health professional.

immunization   the administration, usually by injection, of substances designed to provoke antibodies against specific diseases in order to protect against acquiring these diseases in the future.

immunocompromised   the body's normal defense mechanisms have a decreased ability to respond against disease.

immunosuppresive   an agent that interferes with the body's ability to react to infection.

inflammation   the body's response to trauma or infection, inflammation involves certain special cells and fluids accumulating at the site of injury or infection to help in healing and protecting the area.

insulin   the hormone produced by the pancreas, which is necessary for proper usage of sugar by the body, as well many other important functions.

intravenous (IV)   entering by or occurring within a vein; drugs and fluids are frequently administered intravenously.

lipids   fats normally present in the bloodstream.

menopause   the time of the last menstrual period, associated with a fall in the level of hormone production by the ovaries and sometimes with particular symptoms of this.

methodology   the prescribed techniques by which a test is performed.

neonatal   around the time of birth and the six weeks following birth.

neoplasia   literally "new growth," a term for cancer or precancer.

ophthalmologist   a specialist doctor trained to diagnose and treat all aspects of eye disease.

optometrist   a person trained to assess basic eye function, but not to treat eye disease.

osteoporosis   loss of calcium from the bones, associated with the time after menopause as well as with many other conditions.

ovulation   release of an egg from an ovary.

oxidative stress   changes in the cells due to stressors, such as lack of adequate nutrients that lead to degenerative changes.

oxygen saturation   the percentage of oxygen present in the blood.

pancreas   an organ found behind the stomach which produces insulin and several enzymes necessary for proper digestion.

parathyroid glands   small glands in the neck concerned with calcium regulation in the body.

placenta   the organ attached to a baby in the womb, via the umbilical cord, which nourishes the baby, provides oxygen throughout pregnancy, and removes waste material.

plaque   material like a scab on the interior of blood vessels, composed of cholesterol, cellular debris, and other matter that can lead to blockage of the blood vessels.

pneumococcus   bacteria responsible for some pneumonias and other infections.

polycystic ovary syndrome   a condition in which many small cysts may be present on the ovaries and ovarian hormone production may be abnormal.

polyp   a protuberant growth of skin or other tissue; may develop in many parts of the body; often appears like a cherry on a stalk; may be benign or show cancerous changes.

progestin   synthetic form of the hormone progesterone normally produced by the ovary.

prospective randomized trial   a form of medical testing whereby some individuals are given the drug or product to be tested and others are supplied with a placebo or control substance; the results are accumulated over a period of time during which neither the participants nor those conducting the trial are aware who is receiving the test substance and who is not. Believed to be the most accurate method of assessing medical treatments and drugs.

renal   related to the kidneys.

Rhogam   vaccine given to Rhesus negative women after the birth of a Rhesus-positive baby to prevent the development of antibodies in the mother that could affect future pregnancies

rubella   a viral infection, familiarly called German measles.

serum screen   a test of four blood chemicals during the first four months of pregnancy to screen for Down's syndrome.

sonogram   the pictures taken during an ultrasound examination.

sphygmomanometer   a device consisting of a cuff, pump, and dial that is used to measure blood pressure.

STD   sexually transmitted disease.

stereotactic biopsy   a robotic, or remotely controlled, biopsy directed by ultrasound or X-ray.

transformation zone   the junction of the tissues between the inside and the outside of the cervix; the area from which Pap smears are taken.

T-score   the bone density score derived by comparing the results of an individual's DXA exam to a norm based on young women.

ultrasonometry   the study of organs using medical ultrasound.

unconjugated estriol   a hormone, a type of estrogen, produced by the placenta.

ureters   the tubes connecting the bladder with the kidneys.

uterus   the womb.

Z-score   the bone density score derived by comparing the results of a woman's DXA exam to a norm based on an average of women of the same age.

Further Reading

American Medical Association. *The American Medical Association Complete Medical Encyclopedia.* New York: Random House, 2003.

Beers, Mark, ed. *The Merck Manual of Medical Information: The World's Most Widely Used Medical Reference Now in Everyday Language.* 2d ed. New York: Simon and Schuster, 2003.

Boston Women's Health Collective. *Our Bodies Ourselves for the New Century: A Book for and by Women.* New York: Touchstone Books, 1998.

Gotto, Antonio, ed. *The Cornell Illustrated Encyclopedia of Health: The Definitive Home Medical Reference.* New York: Lifeline Press, 2002.

Index

About the Authors

Michele Moore, M.D., author of *The Only Menopause Guide You'll Need,* is a family physician specializing in women's health. Caroline M. de Costa, M.D., a professor of obstetrics and gynecology at James Cook University School of Medicine, Queensland, is a mother of seven who has undergone a hysterectomy. Moore and de Costa are coauthors of *Do You Really Need Surgery? A Sensible Guide to Hysterectomy and Other Procedures for Women.*